THE ETHICS
OF GENETIC CONTROL

JOSEPH FLETCHER

The Ethics
of Genetic Control
ENDING REPRODUCTIVE ROULETTE

ANCHOR BOOKS
Anchor Press/Doubleday
Garden City, New York
1974

ISBN: 0-385-08257-6
Library of Congress Catalog Card Number 73–81430
Copyright © 1974 by Joseph Fletcher
All Rights Reserved
Printed in the United States of America
First Edition

CONTENTS

FOREWORD   *Joshua Lederberg*

Dilemmas about new knowledge, especially about our own bodies, touch deep-rooted anxieties about man's perception of himself and of the gods that he invents or are revealed to him. Mary Shelley, who created Dr. Frankenstein, subtitled her own work *The New Prometheus*, as witness to a mythical link that spans more than two millenniums. Most of her successors are pale imitators: No great wit is needed to fantasize the mad scientist and the unpredictable outcome of his tampering with the forces of nature. And it is a story line that always sells.

Far harder is it to address the problems of new uses of biology, as Joseph Fletcher does here, in a reality-oriented fashion that exposes the underlying problems of human values. Today instead of Dr. Frankenstein we have physicians and scientists who have dedicated their energies to the relief of disease. The "natural" outcome of a bad hand of genetic cards, or of many other of life's mishaps and misfortunes, is a level of pain and distress that cries out for artificial relief; just as we build fires and weave clothing to keep out nature's chills. And we must learn how not to burn or suffocate ourselves in the process. To outlaw fire may not be man's best path—although Dr. Fletcher reminds us how Prometheus was indeed punished for defying the gods' interdiction. In his plays, Aeschylus tested his fellow Athenians' ethical convictions with far greater authenticity than we can experience from most contemporary debate about technological progress. With his even temper and honest exposure of the premises of his ethical arguments, Dr. Fletcher sets a new standard—and one hopes a precedent for further debate.

Dr. Fletcher comments how quickly things change. Indeed, this book may already be overtaken by changes in the process of science and the bases for its public support that are taking place right now. The fifties and early sixties were a time when the United States was especially conscious of science in the aftermath of Sputnik. Then one might have argued that knowledge in some branches of genetics was doubling every two years. The climate is very different today. National policy makers insist that we already have an excess of scientists and refuse to support training more Ph.D.s; they question long-term needs for more doctors. Research budgets have plateaued, and in some fields the dollar levels are more than overtaken by inflation. Demographic predictions point to a shrinkage of demand for higher education, and with this in the number of places needed for teacher-investigators at the universities.

Real concerns for the welfare of human subjects and a mania for bureaucratic regulation of research in the drug industry are also tempering the rate of advance. In particular it is no longer true that there is a negligible time lag between "the theoretically possible and the clinically feasible." On the contrary, for some drugs, that lag may be as long as ten or fifteen years, with many opportunities for afterthoughts, changes of standards, and the discovery of adverse information that may prolong that lag indefinitely. Whether or not public policy is sounder for this tempering of new introductions, it is certain that we are entering a new phase of built-in resistance to innovation in many spheres.

Some of the more irrational components of this reaction may have been softened if Dr. Fletcher's wisdom had been more widely available sooner. At the moment of this writing, the California state legislature is acting on bills to prohibit research on human fetuses, and the U. S. House of Representatives has already passed such a bill with such an amendment added on the floor. The subject may well be worthy of legislative attention; my complaint is that these bodies have refused to hold open hearings to discuss the complex sets of values that may be at stake. In the wave of emotion, language may become law that includes such phrases as would prohibit "conception outside the womb," as if a test tube could be pregnant.

The most insidious features of these laws is how they imply that experimentation is inherently suspect. They would explicitly forbid certain acts if done for experimental purposes that the law would not touch if done out of malice, or for profit, or for entertainment! Whatever principles underlie these prospective laws, they are a far cry from the existential ethics that Dr. Fletcher advocates. There is of course a political explanation. The public's existential concern for its own welfare and happiness has been expressed on the abortion issue, against the deep-felt convictions of a religious minority. Experimental observations on fetuses can be a symbolic sacrifice to those minority convictions without touching the immediate interests of more than a few investigators. The long-term costs of denying to society the medical information that might be gained by studies on fetuses—including possible ways to treat fetal disease that might result in healthier babies, and the avoidance of some abortions that are now inevitable—these are too remote and too arcane to be widely understood.*

Besides these laws, which focus on experimentation itself, many other social controls limit what can be done on the course of research. The investigator has no license to invade the security of other persons or their property. Besides the informal sanctions that we call common decency, he must, like every other citizen, respect laws on criminal assault and civil recourse to damages for injury. Although a few citizens are thieves, most of us are not obliged to prove in advance that we are innocent of stealing; increasingly, investigators are facing a presumption of guilt, and the demand for more elaborate procedures to prove their innocence.

It is true that a researcher who is also a physician may be in conflict about his obligations to his patients —whose health is his primary obligation. In practice, research already exposes a doctor to special liability for malpractice suits in the event of harm. Even so, legislators can point to unredressed abuses that may justify still more elaborate procedures to protect the rights of uninformed and unconsenting patient-subjects. At the present time, even verbal psychological inquiries that would go unquestioned if done for commercial or

---

* Furthermore, any steps that will make the medical observation of the fetus criminally suspect might help to influence public attitudes in favor of rehabilitating the civil status of the fetus even at the expense of its mother. Advocates of this status, who call themselves "for life," should ponder on the quality of life that would result if genetically damaged fetuses were in fact given legal privileges to exist. We would face the moral obligation of active steps to salvage innumerable creatures whose nurture would be an intolerable burden to themselves, their families, and the social order. It should be more widely known that one fourth of all conceptions now abort spontaneously, but could in principle be saved to protect the right to life of the worst of nature's mishaps.

for administrative purposes must be formally justified before review panels. In many instances these require certificates of the subjects' consent, before they can be pursued in a university research program. These are important instruments of social control of experimentation (contra many assertions that these do not exist); and they must be kept in mind in forecasts about the rate and directions by which fundamental new biological knowledge can be developed *in man*, and applied to *human* problems.

Dr. Fletcher takes care to point out that the time frame is unimportant, that many ethical problems are very properly introduced by the phrase "just suppose." There is much argument among biologists about the time frame in which the developments he discusses will become tangible realities, when their application to man poses individual ethical or aggregate social problems of decision. I agree about the value of the metaphor "just suppose"; but when this is not understood we may have a panic reaction to fantasied urgencies, of which legislation intended to prohibit studies on the human egg is an evident example. My personal prophetic intuition agrees with the foresight of many new opportunities for applying biological science; but the experience of the last two decades suggests that the most important applications will come from entirely new directions, most of them now foreseen and quite different from the Frankenstein's monsters that are painted today. For example, even ten years ago, hardly anyone would have predicted that prenatal diagnosis of disease would develop to the status it now enjoys, while many people were already science-fictionizing about genetic surgery and cloning, which are still speculations.

The boldness of Dr. Fletcher's thinking is to be seen in the directness with which he develops concrete, moral principled answers to many of the dilemmas we can easily spin. This is terribly important, whether or not we agree with his basic ethical principles, for he has exposed these for all to see. There will be conflict about these; much less about the inexorable logic by which he draws humane conclusions—for humane-ity is his logic. His liberality of outlook will inspire many demoralized and confused people, especially parents who have been beset by doubts as to their responsibilities to themselves and to their hoped-for children. He has wise counsels also for many people who in one way or another are involved in biological research and in medical care, and whose technical expertise confers unavoidable moral responsibilities. Those who disagree will at the very least be challenged to re-examine their fundamental beliefs about the validity of moral imperatives that have been invented for man, and which are sometimes in conflict with common-sense measures based on human pain and delight.

My admiration for Dr. Fletcher's work does not, of course, imply that I agree unswervingly about many of the complex issues he has raised here. I have my doubts that we can always measure the human well-being that should be the touchstone of our efforts. Human self-evaluation of right and wrong, of pleasure and pain, is not always autonomous, but itself developed within a social ethos—else why would others persist so passionately in what appears to us to be wrong thinking! Should we not encourage children to defer immediate gratification for the sake of higher pleasures and rewards? In the framework of the social contract, we may all get more freedom by sacrificing some. Can we be oblivious to another's self-injury in contexts like drug abuse or motorcycling without a helmet, without at the same time becoming more callous about their welfare and resenting having to share the medical bills?

The utilitarian principle itself must respect absolute restraints to avoid the tyranny of the majority: For example, we cannot ethically exploit a few people, without their consent, for high risk medical experiments, simply because of the great benefits to the many. It is impossible, then, in my view to avoid some categorical imperatives; but I am with Dr. Fletcher in demanding that we start, rather than finish, our ethical inquiries from such principles; and that, above all, it is the human consequences by which we must judge our acts.

AUTHOR'S NOTE

For 150 years and longer ethicists or, if you prefer, moral philosophers have cited Immanuel Kant's four fundamental questions: What can I know? What ought I to do? What can I hope? What is man? This book is about these questions, especially the second one—the moral question. The other questions, however, are fully involved. Although science can help us with all of them it cannot by itself answer any of them.

Both morality and ethics are face to face with new problems posed by recent startling discoveries in modern biology and genetics in general and in human reproduction in particular. To avoid language confusion and keep out of the semantic swamp we should be clear at the outset that "morality" is what people believe to be right and good, and the reasons they give for it, while "ethics" is critical reflection about morality and the rational analysis of it. We often use the two terms interchangeably and no great harm comes from it, but to be quite precise a *moral* question is, for example, "Should this pregnancy be terminated?" while the *ethical* problem would be, "How shall we go about deciding such a question?"

Advances in reproductive medicine and genetics are so breathtaking that their speed blurs and erodes the distinction between what can be done today and may be done tomorrow. As we shall see, there is a difference between what is and what will be or might be, yet the difference is very fleeting and for ethical or moral purposes it is of little importance. Moral thinking about right and wrong has always dealt with questions by asking "Just suppose." Hypothetical questions are a common stock in the ethics trade: "What should we do if . . ."

In science-based affairs, especially those of a biological kind like medicine, the hypothetical quickly becomes the actual. Future questions foreseen are suddenly present and pressing. The time lag is negligible between the theoretically possible and the clinically feasible. It is said that prophecy foreshortens time, that it treats what is to come as if it were a present fact. In this sense prophecy is a major part of biomedical ethics in these days.

Our traditional morality of baby making is based on heterosexual intercourse or coital conception, and on uterine gestation or fetal nurture in the human womb. This has been superseded or at least become supersedable. Since mores and values always change as conditions and situations change, our morality will and should change too.

For example, moral responsibility (response ability) in human reproduction may be shifted from the simple matter of controlling the number of children we have to the trickier business of controlling the genetic or physical *quality* of our children. It would be quite a jump to go from the blind chances of sexual roulette or "taking what you get" in baby making to the careful production of prefabricated babies. There are other possibilities. Our notion of avarice may have to be broadened to condemn the *selfishness* of keeping our sperm and ova to ourselves exclusively. Justice may come to mean not having large families. Arrogance might be charged against those who wish to produce children in their own image.

Our conventional view of baby making was shaped in an age when we were helplessly ignorant of how to prevent or correct horrors like idiocy or the fatal convulsions of Tay-Sachs disease. In a lighter vein, think of the moral change of pace for a lot of people when they hear that keeping pregnant women booze happy by injecting alcohol into their vascular system holds off labor contractions in some cases for the sake medically of both the mother and the child. This kind of critical revision in our moral attitudes is the job of ethics.

The Cornell physiologist Robert Morison puts it this way:

> There are several reasons for believing that we can no longer keep our system of moral values and our system of scientific expertise in separate water-tight compartments. Perhaps most important is the fact that science, and especially biological science, has produced evidence to reinforce some ancient exhortations and weaken the hold of others, and has invented, or at least called attention to the significance of, an entirely new range of good and bad behavior.[1]

This way of looking at moral problems carries undeniable force now that *for the first time in the evolution of life a living creature (man) has both the understanding and the ability to design itself and its future.* This will "blow our minds" figuratively if not literally. Take gout, for example. It is the only form of arthritis for which we know the cause but up to the present we could only treat it—not prevent it. But at last genetic engineering, so called, aims at preventing it. The disease comes from a defect of the genes and by controlling the genes we could obviate the disease. The redesign of people is taking shape on the biological drawing boards.

In this book, however, there will be no simple or slavish idea that just because something is scientifically (that is, biologically) possible it is therefore good and desirable. My personal conviction, from the vantage point of nearly seventy years of experience, is that Hume was correct: There is no way by logic or sound reasoning to get from an is statement to an ought statement. Facts are one thing, values another. We do not have to like or accept something just because it is possible or even probable. Therefore underneath what follows in this book will be an assumption like Jacques Monod's that wisdom "prohibits any confusion of value judgments with judgments arrived at through knowledge."[2] Statements about what is cannot yield statements about what ought to be. Just because something is a fact or could become a fact does not mean necessarily that it is good or right.

On the other hand, neither is the mere fact that people like or dislike a thing enough to establish it as right or wrong ethically. We ought not to confuse the ethical with the popular. To do so is the essence of conventionalism, the cake of custom; it tends to base ethical judgments simply on opinion polls. For example, in a Harris poll in 1969 it was found that only 21 per cent favored genetics as a way to improve human beings as a species or to produce superior children, but 58 per cent favored the use of genetics in uterine diagnosis to help correct the defects in a particular individual fetus. Men were more opposed than women to the new birth technologies—let women please take note. Yet a majority of both men and women rejected the notion that the new methods are morally wrong.

Now none of these findings settles anything except the is question, assuming that they are accurate. It is said that morally we live under two kinds of ethical influence: the respected opinion maker and the public opinion poll. The first is truly ethics—it is somebody's reasoning about what ought to be. But the second is only reportage, about what is. The real ethical question is "What are we to think, how are we to form a judgment?" Ethics is a jump from the indicative to the normative. George Gallup and Louis Harris are nose counters and tabulators, and that is all. They only tell us factually what people say when questions are put to them by clipboard carriers. The ethical task, however, is to critically analyze the answers given.

Certainly we need more knowledge and fresh thinking, and they are not easy to come by. *The New Yorker* once complained,

> These are hard times for the layman. He is no longer thought competent to work out his own opinions on many matters, even many that touch him intimately. His very survival has become the property of committees and the subject of learned argument among specialists. He has little to say in the affair, poor fish, being largely ignorant of the information upon which plans for him are based.[3]

It is next to impossible for the ordinary person to keep up with the growth of modern knowledge. Science in general has been doubling its information every ten years, biology every five, and genetics every *two* years. Therefore when René Dubos says that we must have "criticism of science formulated by enlightened nonscientists"[4] the real problem is one of getting the nonscientists enlightened. When Sir Peter Medawar declares, "It is absolutely right that the public should scrutinize the activities of physicians and scientists . . . and unconditionally necessary that we should make them understand,"[5] it follows that books like this one are very much in order.

Science and technology are the precipitators of most of our moral questions. As they add to our knowledge and thus to our control and power of choice, they frequently pose new issues about right and wrong, good and evil, desirable and undesirable. Or, as is often the case, old issues are raised in new forms. In human reproduction, for example, ethical problems of the sort examined in this book are a result of medicine's success, not of its failure. Very likely it will be harder to succeed with the ethical problems than with the medical problems, since a lot more human feeling and conflicting attitudes will be involved once these issues "go public."

A great many able people have contributed descriptive or journalistic studies of genetics and the new reproductive biology, in a nontechnical or popular way: Taylor, Rosenfeld, Leach, Francoeur, Augenstein, Comfort, Still, Rorvik, Warshofsky. It makes an imposing roster. But inevitably these books have repeated each other and to some extent rewashed the same laundry. They have pointed to pretty much the same moral questions, as questions without answers. We are spinning our wheels. Reading nearly all the journals along with more popular media I find that people are saying the same things and asking the same questions over and over.

What, then, can excuse still another one—this one? My answer is that this one tries to give some answers, not just ask the questions. It makes the jump or leap from the indicative to the normative. It tries to be analytic, not merely descriptive; unlike the others it tackles the facts evaluatively, ethically; it attempts (uneasily yet not too timidly) to move on from the is side to the ought side. Obviously it will not and cannot once and for all "wrap up" the ethical issues, but hopefully it may help.

Two or three little books more or less on these questions have appeared from special religious or theological points of view. They too will come in for attention as we go along. However, the reader should know right away that *this* book is written from a humanistic perspective; it is not religious and does not claim to have any knowledge of God's will beyond the conviction that any God worth believing in wills the best possible well-being for human beings. This is what the Bible calls love, concern for persons. Under this standard or ideal there ought not to be any significant practical difference in the ethical judgments of either theological or humanistic inquirers.

With the weakening of authoritarian ethics morality is being based more and more pragmatically on human need and less and less on alleged revelations of the divine will or arguments based on such revelations. If we are concerned with ethical realism we should welcome this trend. It is a desirable advance in mental and moral humility, in a free world of pluralistic moral judgment. Our criterion or ideal, then, will be what is humane and rational, not what is revealed or authoritarian.

As Henry Miller, vice-chancellor of the University of Newcastle, has pointed out: "The reason for a moral code is pragmatic . . . The scientist's approach to morals is utilitarian. The fact that it quite often happens to coincide with the attitudes of Christianity indicates that even the most improbable of religions has to keep its feet on the ground if it is to remain relevant."[6]

We have gone through so many "ages" of late: the Atomic Age, the Electronic Age, the Space Age—and now the Biotic Age. This may be a strange term but it will soon be quite familiar. After the First World War and the revolutions that went with it in the twenties we were all focused ethically on the social sciences. Then came a shift of attention to the behavioral sciences and the questions posed by psychology. Next, with the Second World War and the atomic breakthrough, we had to cope with a new set of ethical issues due to the physical sciences. Now we are faced (it all moves so fast) with even more challenging and worrisome moral problems of a still newer kind, along the biological front. Invading the secrets of the atom's nucleus never raised moral questions any more imperative than those that face us in the genetic invasion of the human cell's nucleus.

We will be exploring and finding answers which are sure to cut across the conventional wisdom. Our task is to avoid falling for scary horror stories on the one hand and, on the other, to avoid smugly glossing over the risks and the costs. Unhappily both of these reactive ploys are altogether too common.

Every innovation raises at least a few hackles. A case in point is the practice of artificial insemination, which got its start under cover of secrecy as far back as 1890 in the work of Dr. Robert L. Dickinson. As a distinguished specialist in New York put it recently, people greeted artificial insemination first with horror, then rejection, then curiosity, followed by more study and finally by acceptance.[7] William James found the same pattern in the reception given to his pragmatism. First they said, "Nonsense. It's absurd." Then it changed to, "Obvious. A platitude." At last they said, "Very true. And very important. This is what I've been saying all along."

I have tried throughout and conscientiously to avoid loaded language. Argument is loaded necessarily and legitimately, but what the biologist Garrett Hardin calls "blackwashing" terms (like whitewashing) ought to be out of bounds. Psychosemantic reinforcements, such as talking about "little unborn babies" in the abortion debate, usually boomerang on their employers anyway.

Without their being at all accountable for what I say, I have learned a lot from such eminent physicians and biologists as the Nobel laureate Joshua Lederberg, Louis Lasagna, Garrett Hardin, René Dubos, Conrad Waddington, Jean Rostand, Henry Beecher, Van Potter, Dwight Ingle, Edmund Pellegrino, Theodosius Dobzhansky, Bentley Glass. There are so many. My very real personal thanks are due to the steadying counsel of my colleague in the Human Biology and Society Program, Dr. Thomas Harrison Hunter, and others of our colleagues in the University of Virginia's School of Medicine, to the Commonwealth Fund for its support, to Mary Burke Wagner for her efficient help in research and office management, and to my wife, Forrest, not only for her unflagging interest but her clear-eyed and clear-headed comments as the book took shape.

Finally, my gratitude to Dr. Joshua Lederberg can hardly be put in words. A mere layman both in scientific and medical matters, my work would have been even more amateurish than it is without his personal interest and criticism. Except in matters of fact I have sometimes risked taking my own line, but even so his corrective comments have been of immeasurable help and strength. He and my other colleagues are hereby exculpated from any involvement in my errors or ignorances. Where I am right, thank them; where I am wrong, blame me.

Charlottesville, Virginia, and   Joseph Fletcher
Belmont, Massachusetts

I

SOME IDEAS

Our habit is to think of the compassionate Prometheus himself when we say something is "Promethean." That brave son of a Titan was inspired by his concern for the miseries of men to steal fire from heaven for their use, thus enraging Zeus.

Even Webster's gives this meaning. But in truth the etymology of the word is what is important, not its hero nor his mythology. Prometheus comes from *pro* and *mathein*, to learn or think beforehand or ahead of time. It means forethought—which is what this book is all about.

We hear a lot these days about futurology. Bertrand de Jouvenal thinks we ought to call it futuristics because "ology" suggests that information is already at hand when, by definition, any attempt to foretell or foresee the future has to get along without the future's data. Alvin Toffler's *Future Shock* has done more than anything else by a social analyst to alert the general public to the need of prudently anticipating trends, policies, and decisions as well as we can. Toffler refers to "the biological witches' brew" and says, "The moral and emotional choices that will confront us in the coming decades are mind-staggering."[1]

Occasionally the man in the street hears something about probing the future when environmentalists warn us about the danger of exhausting our natural resources, or when a Daniel Ellsberg exposes the Pentagon Papers secretly used by the Rand Corporation's "think tank" for war contingency planning, or when Herman Kahn offers us some "thinking about the unthinkable" from his Hudson Institute. Yet the trouble in all of this is that we persist in assuming that the future will somehow resemble the past—even in our planning—*and this is wrong.*

But do we really take at all seriously the imperative need to try our best to look into the future? And in making decisions and policy choices, as they affect our own lives individually as well as the collective affairs of mankind, do we realize that some of the choices we make are irreversible—and will be more so, increasingly? In Dennis Gabor's phrase, "The future cannot be predicted, but futures can be invented."[2] At the same time, however, the chains of consequences following from some of our innovations and decision making are of such a radical nature that we cannot "go back again" to the fork in the road, to take the other road instead, no matter how much we might wish we could.

For example, there is no going back on the decision to split and fuse atoms; that fierce fire, for good or for evil, has been snatched from the gods (that is, from our former ignorance), and there is no giving it back. We have lost our innocence and left the Garden of Eden, that mythic past situation which seems so ideal and safe to those for whom ignorance is bliss. Yearning after Arcadia, the perfect past state, is as irrelevant to the realities of human existence as yearning for Utopia, the perfect future state.*

---

* Sir Thomas More distinguished between U-topia, an imaginary country that does not exist, and Eu-topia, a country which could be real as well as ideal. But Utopia in our ordinary use (the second meaning) is as unlikely as the first.

Well, just as the technology of nuclear power is on an irreversible, world-shaking course, so the discovery of behavior controls and molecular and cellular biology's grasp of how to design or alter the genetic constitution of human beings might well be not only man shaking but irreversible, at least in some of their uses. Storied explorations of the past were really small potatoes compared to the potential importance of present-day scientific explorations, especially the biological revolution and its new birth technologies.

The biological revolution is a quantum or dialectical leap in human change. It is an instance of what Marx and his cohort Engels tried to explain as the "transformation of quantity into quality."

Sanitation and preventive medicine have already raised the quantity of people (with some serious dangers resulting as undesired side effects); now, as a new turn in our affairs, we are at last in a position biologically to increase the *quality* of the babies we make. All of this adds up to what Joshua Lederberg calls "orthobiosis"—setting things right by applying the life sciences. The most elemental changes are not going on in the external or material world but in the minds and flesh of human beings. In the order of revolution the biologists are outdoing the Presidents and Parliaments and Pentagons.

We sometimes hear the objection and warning that genetic selection and engineering would rule out geniuses because geniuses often have serious things wrong with them. (The same argument is used against therapeutic or eugenic abortion.) A common ploy along this line is to ask, "Do you want to lose Beethoven just to get rid of his deafness?" This is only tricky illogic. If we can weed out Beethoven's deafness, let's do it. He was a great composer and pianist in spite of his defect, not because of it. Dostoevski's literary gifts were not due to his epilepsy. Wagner was a psychopath *and* a great musician; there was no cause and effect relation between the two things. The intention of genetic engineering is to locate and alter the genes which cause defects in superior people. The idea is to get rid of the bad traits in order to liberate the good ones.

Discoveries like genetic coding make the breakthroughs of the old-fashioned hard technologies seem like child's play.[3] It is at least arguable that genetics and artificial reproduction, with all of their moral entanglements, are more important advances than fire, printing, and the wheel have been. Jean Rostand and others say that *homo sapiens* is becoming *homo biologicus*. But not so. It is precisely because men are sapient that they can control their biology. If we like word play it would be better to speak of *homo autofabricus*.

This book will hold our focus on genetics and human reproduction but the full range open to *homo autofabricus* might be seen in a side glance at decisions going on about interspecific hybrids, man-animal hybrids.[4] Biological research has shown that genes are genes; they can combine across species lines. Desirable roles and functions for chimeras or humanoids can be imagined. If human females reject copulation with, for example, a pongid (high primates such as chimpanzees, gorillas, and orangs) hybridization could be done by artificial insemination or by fertilization *in vitro*, followed by implantation of the embryo in a human, pongid, or artificial womb. If this was unacceptable a pongid female could be inseminated or implanted, to do the gestating. If neither method proved possible or desirable it could be done by implanting an embryo in a glass womb for artificial gestation to birth. Bizarre certainly, repellent to some, but it spells out the radical character of the new frontier.

A warning or caution is in order at this early point. Having babies is not necessarily the greatest thing in the world. For some it has a number-one priority, for others it may be no part of their scheme of things. In some cases it is undesirable even if they want it: genetic deformity and disease, neglect and child abuse, parental inadequacy even with a good will—these are some of the realities which support the ethics of biological selection and control. There are very good reasons to oppose any uncritical claim to the "right" to reproduce.

In any case women are not baby machines and men are not seedcasters. Explaining how we can have babies in many different ways is not beating the drum for making babies. Our bias is for fewer babies and better ones, whether they are made naturally or in the new artificial modes. In the so-called vaginal politics of the women's liberation we have a very sound stance morally.

René Dubos is right to claim that the future is humankind's own creation as much as it is the result of circumstances, and that man now has the "privilege and the responsibility of shaping his self" as well as his future.[5] Beyond any precedent we are now in a position to change not only the social and environmental conditions of mankind but even man himself, his very stuff.

At the same time, as we face up to our new powers, we should try to avoid two ethical errors that lurk near at hand. One is the capacity fallacy, the notion that because we can do something, such as genetic control, we ought to. It does not follow that because we could we should. The other error is the necessity fallacy, the assumption of inevitability—that because we can do something we *will*. For those who are governed by this kind of fatalism this book's look into the ethical issues is only a waste of time.

As a matter of fact there is a third related fallacy, the growth fallacy—a simplistic notion that "more is good." We can see how this idea in the case of population has jeopardized the quality of life in many respects. Many of the consequences of technological growth, pollution for example, are so destructive or so great a nuisance that we are beginning to rediscover the law of diminishing returns; progress with a capital "P" is called into question.

To put it more carefully, we are recognizing that increase does not equal progress. John Stuart Mill's model of the stationary or equilibrium state is being dusted off again, and if the cost-benefit balance rightly applies to advances in the hard technology of industry it can also apply to the soft technology of medical care. This is not said, of course, to discourage our increase of control over the quality of human beings. But it does mean that every advance proposed ought to be scrutinized carefully in terms of the values we strive to preserve or achieve. It is precisely this which an ethical critique of the new reproductive biology is trying to do.

Our situation is Promethean. We are "trying to play God," as some say. Looked at from another point of view, we are adding to our knowledge and control of our human condition. This takes us far beyond anything we once believed to be within the range of human powers. At the same time we therefore have much more reason to try as imaginatively as we can to foresee the consequences of "stealing such powers from the gods"—and not only the immediate but the remote consequences. We have to look ahead; futuristics is, we might say, the modern practice of the ancient virtue of prudence.

Winston Churchill used to grumble that it is always wise to look ahead but difficult to look farther than you can see. It was easier to solve cleaning problems as we did with detergents than it was to foresee that pollution would follow. Yet this two-sidedness is always the case with our decisions and policy choices, and when the unknown future figures in as well as the known past it is easy to see how uncertainly the best of intentions can work out. Nostradamus, they say, had a plaque on his wall which read: "It is very difficult to prophesy, especially about the future."

The Biotic Age

We are on the first lap of a biological revolution, with all the promise and the threat that great revolutions carry. James D. Watson, codiscoverer with Francis Crick of the DNA "double helix," which is the key to living organisms, told a House committee in Washington in 1971 that *in vitro* (test tube) methods of reproduction will be routine in ten to twenty years, and that "cloning" or reproduction from one parent only (using a body cell instead of combining a sperm and ovum) will be an accomplished fact in twenty to twenty-five years, if not sooner. Arthur Kornberg, another Nobel laureate, says we may get weary of the label "revolutionary" but nothing else fits what has happened in biomedical exploring.[6] On the other hand, of course, what has happened is not a sudden or inexplicable break with "normalcy" but a big jump forward in a steady movement toward converting the dark and ominous secrets of biological life into lighted and manageable reality. Revolutions are only stages in evolution when the rate of change is abnormally rapid.

Most scientists, especially physicians, are considered to be conservative. They are not revolutionaries. Nevertheless, what has emerged in genetics and embryology and fetal control is in fact revolutionary. Man's biological evolution has always moved along with what Bentley Glass once called "glacial slowness."[7] But now in only the past few years, with uncomfortable speed, men have begun to take charge of their own evolution. It was only twenty years ago that one of the first textbooks on medical genetics was published and promoted in an advertising campaign among doctors, and it was a miserable failure. There were hardly any sales.

We are moving away from accidental and toward directed mutation in the basic structures of human individuals, by means of X rays, lasers, high-speed electrons, neutrons, or alpha particles. Insect societies are stable (stagnant?) for millennia because they are shaped by genetic transmission over which insects have no control. Unlike the locked-in bugs, men are at last able creatively to shape their own lives—genetically as well as socially and culturally.

Teilhard de Chardin put it in an exciting and characteristic way: Men, he said, are now in a position fully to "seize the tiller of the world." Julian Huxley once remarked that "man now finds himself in the unexpected position of business manager for the cosmic process of evolution." As recently as Newton, Darwin, and Mendel, biology was still a study of nature's processes in order to understand how nature works, but in the twentieth century there has been a conversion of the scientific motive from "just to know" to "how to control with what we know."

Postconception, prenatal control, is possible now

with aseptic and medically safe abortion, and by intrauterine genetic diagnosis along with fetal surgery and medication. And finally, when genetic surgery and therapy reach at last the goals already on their drawing boards we will have control over the quality of the infants to be born even *before* conception. Yet this is all so new that no existing "code" of medical ethics has any ground rules at all for the research needed on fetal tissue or germ plasm, nor for the use of what we are finding out.

All of this means we have entered upon positive or *direct* eugenic control, and that we have surmounted the inadequacy and errors of negative control by selective mating. At least we have added positive to negative means. A hundred years ago Sir Francis Galton was inspired by his cousin Charles Darwin's *On the Origin of Species* to propose control of our genetic quality by selecting our mates, choosing them for their physical and mental qualities rather than just taking "potluck" with sheerly impulsive romance.

The whole scheme depended, however, on some dubious ideas about which traits are transmissible in the germ plasm. The "eugenics movement" had a simplistic notion if not actually a mechanistic one about the correlation between personal qualities and the genetic process. A good way to see the point is found in the story about George Bernard Shaw. When somebody proposed that he father a baby with Isadora Duncan to unite his high intelligence with her great beauty he replied, "No. The poor child might have my looks and her brains."

In this new biotic age our human fortunes are far more influenced by those we might call "intranauts" than by the astronauts.[8] These explorers of the inner spaces of man are the biochemists, immunologists, embryologists, placentologists, teratologists, geneticists, fetologists, and so on. They are much more important in our lives and we are affected far more by their discoveries than by what mere moon walkers and rock collectors do for us. Yet even the intranauts' labels and language are unfamiliar, while the astronauts' lingo is on the front pages. The public has been catching up only very slowly with the meaning of organ transplants, antibiotics, mechanical organ valves and pumps, artificial tissues, myoelectric prostheses (artificial limbs), machine supports such as kidney dialysis, respirators, and pacemakers, chemotherapy, transistorized electronic monitors, and cryonics.

Now on top of all this comes the newest frontier—birth technologies and genetic controls. These controls operate all the way from the germ cell through fertilization and gestation and fetal control to the delivery and postnatal therapy of newborns. Biology has come a long way from being merely that old-fashioned "natural history" which but a short time ago was a fit subject, as Taylor has reminded us, mainly for "young ladies and elderly clergymen."[9]

The quip heard in corner bars is quite soundly based: We first found out how to have sex without babies, and now we are finding out how to have babies without sex. No longer is human reproduction centered in the genitalia or even dependent on them. Even the gonads, testicles and ovaries are no longer necessary. In fact, we have bypassed in theory even the "gametes" or germ cells (eggs and sperm) supplied by the gonads, since theoretically they can be artificially synthesized—that is, constructed chemically without the biological process of forming them.

The age-old saying *omnes vivum ex ovo*, all life comes from the egg, simply is not true any longer. We now understand how to produce by "cloning" a new individual from a body cell—either male or female. The ancient Israelite Abraham laughed at the suggestion that he at one hundred and his wife at ninety could produce a child. She did it by a miracle or divine favor, in the Genesis story, but nowadays, as we shall see, it could be managed in a number of different ways, without any supernatural assists. Even though some of this new capability is not yet in the clinic, the mere knowledge of it irreversibly alters our feelings, attitudes, and meanings.

The question in James Thurber and E. B. White's classic *Is Sex Necessary?* was a joke in innocence in 1929, but now the answer is definitely No. Now we know. Sex in the sense of coital intercourse is no longer necessary for human reproduction. "Where do babies come from?" will henceforth have to be very differently answered, even to children. In 1931, Aldous Huxley in *Brave New World* predicted that "test tube" baby making would come in six hundred years. Actually it is here now as far as conception goes, and it may be that less than twenty-five years will find us managing to bring fetal growth to term in glass wombs. "The prophecies made in 1931 are coming true much sooner than I thought they would," he said in *Brave New World Revisited* (1958). The same is true of the babies we will make; chemistry and surgery will alter the basic genetic construction of the babies we make. No longer will "It's inherited" be a formula of resignation or a reason for despair.

Medicine's rate of discovery is on an exponential course. As a former surgeon general once said, "One discovery opens twenty doors," meaning that our knowledge like our population grows geometrically, not just arithmetically. Furthermore, the rate of growth gets extra leaps along the way from serendipity, unsought and unexpected discoveries which pop up like extra dividends on hard work and curiosity. The X ray resulted from a chance encounter between a metal key and some film on a lab bench; penicillin came from an open window and a breeze blowing loose a pile of mold in another laboratory.

The Taste for Ignorance

At the same time ('twas ever thus) some people react to all of this with "fear and trembling." While Kierkegaard used this phrase to express humility, re-actionaries actually do fear and tremble. They look upon genetic and fetal control with horror, seeing in it only the specter of Mad Scientists and a Huxleian-Hitlerian dictatorship over a human ant heap. But probing by such means as *in vitro* cultures of blasto-cysts (primitive embryos) is important if we are to find out why things go wrong with babies, and how they happen. The investigators doing it "are not perverted men in white coats doing nasty experiments on human beings, but reasonable scientists carrying out perfectly justifiable research."[10]

We are told that we should "let nature alone" and "keep out of the womb" and stop "tinkering" with the building blocks of human beings because we are get-ting "too close to the mystery of life." How close is too close? Why should we not get so close that like other mysteries the secret of life comes to be no secret at all? Robert Sinsheimer of the California Institute of Technology points out that the opponents of ge-netic engineering "aren't among the losers in the chromosomal lottery," which saddles us with "four mil-lion Americans born with diabetes, or the two hundred fifty thousand children born in the United States every year with genetic diseases, or the fifty million Americans whose I.Q.s are below ninety."[11] Genetic engineering and fetal control will help enormously.

The accusation that the new biology is trying to create a "master race" is fair enough if it means that a people with fewer defects and more control over the crippling accidents of "nature" are better able to master life's ups and downs. Most of us would want to belong to the master race in that sense. Mastery in the sense of good health and inheritance is sanity.

Language is a subtle weapon. Terms like "human engineering" and "genetic manipulation" may raise our hackles and usually are meant to. Foot draggers even cry for putting a stop to research and development along these lines, or at least a moratorium, on the ground that it is dangerous knowledge too easily put to evil uses. The finiteness of human knowledge, what C. S. Peirce called "fallibilism," has always motivated some people to try to find answers while it has immobilized and paralyzed others. Science fictioneers, for instance, are sometimes tempted to turn out things like Frederick Pohl's book *The Nightmare Age*, which would make anybody's hair stand on end.†

Since Aldous Huxley's brilliant fable *Brave New World* is constantly mentioned by the scaremongers it should be remembered that Huxley was not (repeat, was not) trying to picture the uses and misuses of biological controls, probable or improbable. Aldous, after all, was a true Huxley; he believed in both biology and democracy. In his fantasy he was setting up a utopia in reverse, or a dystopia, and his aim was political, not cultural; he was warning us against totali-

---

† A far more sophisticated and truly fascinating picture of the future biologically and ethically is Anthony Burgess' *The Wanting Seed* (Ballantine Books), 1963, comparable to the ethical issue he dramatizes in his better known book of the same year, *The Clockwork Orange*.

tarianism, not medical biology, and he decided to use biology only as a major instrument of his imaginary dictatorship. In a new foreword (for the 1946 edition) he pointed out that in his story the dictatorship created the biological nightmare, not the other way around, and that other nonbiological controls could have been used to the same end.

To drive this point home, in his 1958 follow-up essay on the danger of totalitarianism, *Brave New World Revisited*, Huxley foresaw the advent of dictatorship as a likely result of overpopulation (as Burgess does in his *Wanting Seed*). Its system of control, he thought this time, would be one of brainwashing, not of "test tube" baby making. Discussing "What Can Be Done?" he made a strong plea for birth control but said *not a word about suppressing biological science nor even a moratorium on its progress.*

In any case we have no need to look at what is often called "human nature" as either angelic or demonic in order to realize that *dangerous knowledge is not half as dangerous as dangerous ignorance.* The old saw "What you don't know won't hurt you" is dangerous and foolish folk talk. On any sane view of the problem the choice is not between research and know-nothingism but between putting our knowledge to good or to evil uses. In a symposium at Cal Tech Sinsheimer said in an equable spirit, "We have really two choices; to proceed with all the wisdom we can develop, or to stagnate in fear and in doubt. There is a consequence to either choice."[12] Kornberg put it in a nutshell: "Will we stop thinking? Will free men stop wondering? Will people with courage stop building? And if we stop in this country, could we stop people all over the world? . . . You cannot close men's minds all over the world."[13]

The Cassandras and Jeremiahs and Gloomy Guses

are a part of the problem, not of its solution. Technology, whether of the "hard" physical kind or the "soft" biological kind, is man's creation and man's hallmark. We should rejoice, not be ashamed, because norethisterone is used to suspend "monthlies" to let a bride skip a period during her honeymoon or to let an Olympic woman star compete as freely as male athletes do. To be civilized is to be artificial, and to object that something is artificial only condemns it in the eyes of subrational nature lovers or natural-law mystics.

Love making and baby making have been divorced. Sex is free from the contingencies and complications of reproduction, and sexual practice can now proceed on its own merits as an independent value in life. Mary Calderone quotes a doctor's definition of a woman as "a uterus surrounded by a supporting organism and a directing personality."[14] This notion that women are baby machines comes from influences like St. Augustine's; he insisted that sex is only permissible if it aims at or is at least open to conception. The doctrine behind this old morality was that the "end" of intercourse "intended" by nature is reproduction. It has undergirded the antisexual idea that love making on its own merits is sinful, and abortion is murder. This attitude is quite common among doctors of medicine as well as doctors of divinity.

Eastman and Hellman in their twelfth edition of the classic *Williams' Obstetrics* say blandly that pregnancy is "the highest function of the female reproductive system."[15] This canard that pregnancy is normal cultivates the feeling that nonpregnancy is immoral if not actually pathological. Exactly that feeling has been acted out in hospital T.A. (therapeutic abortion) committees, in their automatic ritual of *psychiatric* examination for women seeking to terminate a pregnancy. It raises the interesting question: If she is most truly a woman when she is pregnant, what is she during the other sixty to sixty-five years of her life when she is not pregnant?

Isaac Asimov is quoted as saying, "Babies are the enemies of the human race"—a remark obviously intended to startle us into taking overpopulation seriously.[16] It is often asserted that the Mother of the Year should be a woman who has had a voluntary sterilization and *adopted* two or even three children. "Make love, not people." This is the rock-bottom fact of the new age and the new morality.

The biomedical sciences and arts empower us to improve the quality of our babies and, as a part of our quality control, we shall have to control their numbers. Quality of life depends on the quantity of people trying to live together, their density as well as their physiques and brain makeup. It is almost laughable to recall that Freud, whose nineteenth-century myopia eventually led him into conflict with women's liberation forces because he thought that anatomy is destiny (meaning that women are baby machines), also thought there was no point to medical progress if it did not allow us to have more children. If he had said *better* children instead of more we could take him more seriously. As a result of separating sex and reproduction we now have two functions, not just one, and each must be dealt with on its own merits.

As Dr. Edmund Pellegrino reminds us, a simplistic repetition of the Hippocratic oath ducks moral responsibility; old medical "codes" are at best only statements of ideals needing constant change.[17] Moral sentiments change radically. A schoolmaster in Spandau, Germany, in 1797 was kicked out for publishing a landmark study of plant fertilization; his offense was suggesting that flowers were not entirely sexless, which made him a scandalous detractor from their purity.

Genetics and fetal control will inevitably reorient medicine in a far-reaching way, from the corrective, or curative, to the preventive and re-creative. The appropriate adage is that a stitch in time will save nine.

Keeping Up With the Times

New knowledge forces us uncomfortably to reappraise many things—family relations, life and death, male and female, good and evil, personal identity and integrity, parental ties, health and disease—nearly everything. Also old moral sayings often take on new or added meanings, as with a familiar teaching in the Sermon on the Mount: "Can grapes be picked from briers, or figs from thistles? . . . A good tree cannot bring forth bad fruit, or a poor tree good fruit." That ancient teaching is now an ethical principle with all of the weight of genetics behind it.

But even though biology like psychology can show us how different attitudes or temperaments come about in people, it cannot furnish any reason why we should prefer one attitude to the other. Old Thomas Huxley made the same point long ago. Science with its feats can tilt the ethical table but it cannot settle right and wrong. J. B. S. Haldane explained that a biologist can tell us something about possibilities but never what is worth doing.[18] We can believe that a normal mouth is better than a harelip and that it is better to sense colors than to be color blind, but there is no way biologically to convince anybody that we are right. Santayana was correct; there is no such thing as moral *knowledge*.

Scientific knowledge increases our options and it is well to act with knowledge, yet science is also making our choices steadily more complex and headachy. This is so much so that there is real danger of a "neurologic overload" in both ethics and science. At least it seems that as we are less puzzled or perplexed by the medical problems we are more puzzled and perplexed by the moral problems.

Many people would rather "do" their ethics with the old tried-and-true proverbs and "keep their consciences simple and straightforward" without any of the newfangled and "permissive tricks" of the new morality. But life and culture, i.e., change, are against them. Philosophers, theologians, wisemen—none of them know enough any more to hand down moral *dicta*. They have to consult with biomedical experts. They can ask questions in a kind of catalytic role but they no longer have any prepackaged answers for troubled consciences. The old moralists are ex-moralists.

Alfred North Whitehead and others who have examined human ideas rigorously have concluded that science is indifferent to ethics. They think it is characteristic of science that it ignores all judgments of values, both esthetic and moral. It is true, no doubt, that science as such, according to its own principles, has no morality or ethics except the truth and that its fruits can be used in ways that are both constructive and destructive to human life. But *scientists* are not above or beyond morality and values. Therefore all talk in or out of scientific circles of their work being "value free" is either foolish or knavish. Yet you can search the indexes and tables of content in scientific works on the new biology until your eyes water without finding even the term "ethics," and morality occurs so little it is negligible.

The three questions in ethics concern what we want, how we get it, and why we should. Science cannot settle what we want nor can it explain why we should want it, but when it comes to the *how*, science is the basic source of information. Montaigne held that "science without conscience is but death of the soul." People who are antiscience, strident people who use bad-mouth words such as "scientism," like to quote Montaigne's remark, yet all he meant by it was that lore and learning, whether scientific or humanistic, should serve ethical goals and human welfare. In short, God help us if the sciences are not "done" by humane scientists, and God help us if the humanities are not "done" by scientifically disciplined humanists.

Some people feel that mastery drives out mystery, and that when we dig into nature's secrets, so complicated and yet so simple, we lose our sense of awe and humility. They believe that we should therefore preserve the mystery of birth and baby making by leaving such things alone. This is another form of the Arcadian, Garden of Eden yearning for blissful ignorance. Its expression is often a part of religious piety. When such self-imposed myopia quotes the Gospel of Matthew, "Sufficient unto the day is the evil thereof," we have the exact opposite of this book's future probing and knowledge seeking. Such a passive-dependent sentiment, and indeed that whole passage in the Sermon, is a good example of prescientific, old-world complacency about our future and the knowledge at stake.

Not all religionists take an anti-Promethean posture, however. They occupy a fairly wide spectrum of positions. On the one hand, an official Vatican newspaper once declared that a horse will be able to build an airplane before man has created a living cell. This was said, it is amusing to note, less than a decade before the news came out that Nobelist Gobind Khorana and his associates had succeeded in artificially synthesizing a DNA chain—the basic building block of life.

On the other hand, charitable nuns in Rome contribute their postmenopausal urine to help with FSH fertility research; it is collected daily in a tank truck. FSH is a "follicle stimulating hormone" used in a drug called Pergonal to treat ovaries which do not release enough eggs. It can also be made, but more expensively, from the anterior pituitaries of cadavers. This help from the sisters by the way is an interesting case of the "division of labor," as well as Christian charity, because the nuns have no need of the hormone, being committed to voluntary sterility, while subovulent women wishing for a child and frustrated by inert follicles need the artificial stimulus of the FSH.

One of the most searching and basic issues to take shape in modern times is whether life is a process or something already given and essentially complete. It is an issue which arises whether we are looking at the cosmos, at history, or at human beings. For example, to get right down to the individual, are we to think of life and death as a development on a continuum or are we to see them as events? Biology and medicine know that life does not start with a bang at conception; the life of a person never suddenly pops into being either before or after birth nor does death "happen" at some exact point in time. Life is a continuum or chain or process; so is personality; so is death.

The nineteenth century saw the main battle come to a head between the more or less static "creationist" viewpoint of the prescientific religious and philosophical traditions, and the evolutionary or process viewpoint which took over as the physical and biological sciences progressed.[19] Process philosophy and theology, which understand things to be primarily dynamic rather than static, have no place in them for the conservative or complacent attitude that tends to want moratoriums on theory and practice—to stand still by choice. The fact is we cannot stand still, not even if we want to. Nirenberg by no means sees things through rose-colored glasses yet he states firmly, none-theless, "My guess is that cells will be programmed with synthetic messages within twenty-five years."[20] This is an utterly revolutionary assertion.

We often quote Hamlet, "There are more things in heaven and earth, Horatio, than are dreamt of in your philosophy," and it applies not only because of Horatio's ignorance of what is already to be known but also because of the constantly unfolding reality of life, and our reunderstanding as it unfolds. Today's knowledge is often tomorrow's error. Therefore it is optimism or hope, great expectations, which supply the drive for prophets and revolutionaries. Doomsters and dark viewers cannot be innovators nor can they be happy with life, since it comes up constantly with new and disturbing revelations. Newness is inexorable.

In this process world of ours human life is shaped by three forces especially: First, there is the genetic code which all by itself has been changing only very slowly but may from now on be manipulated into crucial changes for individuals and the species alike; second, there are environmental forces (physical and social) and our adaptive responses—for example, to ecological imperatives; and third, our human capacity to make choices and contrive controls.[21]

Controls are purposive, goal oriented. The over-all social goal is, of course, survival first and improvement second—an increase in whatever values motivate men corporately. Time after time in what follows we shall see how shrewd it was of Gerald Feinberg[22] to list three kinds of control strategies: *divertive*, as when we try to control men's hopes and fears with religion or propaganda; *environmental*, like controlling the biosphere socially and ecologically; and *reconstructive*, to be seen now in the biological control of man's physical structure genetically.

Divertive controls are very ancient as we see in religion's "pie in the sky" but they still take contemporary forms, for example, the drugs route to "inward consciousness." What Feinberg calls the environmental techniques, whether in Marxism's social revolution or the Sierra Club's forest-and-stream gospel, have played a major part in our social struggles. But the newest and strangest kind of goal seeking to emerge is the third kind—the *reconstructive*. This is at the heart of the biological revolution. Its thrust is not toward man's ideology or his world but to reconstruct man himself.‡

Even a religious philosopher and scientist might be willing to endorse the biological revolution, with its human reconstruction of humans. Thus Teilhard de Chardin thought, "So far we have certainly allowed our race to develop at random" but now we should give some thought to "what medical and moral factors must replace the crude forms of natural selection . . ."[23] For this reason the Jesuit paleontologist, whose church at first blacklisted his work, then softened its ban, was convinced that "something is happening in the structure of human consciousness," that "another species of life is just beginning." We do not have to resort to his religious belief in a cosmic "megasynthesis" converging on the "Omega Point" (God) in order to feel the weight of his process viewpoint. In any case we have good reason to see that "the descent of man" (as Darwin titled one of his

‡ Should we drop the generic term "man" and its pronoun "his" and use something like "human beings" and "their" instead? It is probably true that *psychologically* "man" carries a male connotation, even if unconsciously. As we have seen, language is not unimportant.

books) is really the *rise* of man: human evolution is a descent in time but a climb in complexity and capability.

Prudence and Forward Motion

Prudence calls upon us to talk about the biological revolution as much as we can in a low key, to avoid arousing unrealistic expectations and then an unintended backlash. Powerful currents of expectation tend to rise exponentially. Just as every door opened by research unlatches twenty more, so every hope or fear aroused begins to swell like a balloon. It is plain that one important new thing in our time is newness itself; there is a change in the scope of change itself. None of us can any more escape the old Chinese curse "May you live in a time of transition."

Joshua Lederberg told a Senate hearing that in ten to thirty years we could do "essentially anything that we care to do in the area of biological engineering," adding, however, that we are not likely to get there because society will not invest the 10 to 20 per cent of our gross national product required to fund it. Nonetheless, he was sure that our ability to fabricate viruslike agents to correct some gene defects is a "virtual certainty well within a decade."[24] Lederberg is a man of humility, not of arrogance. What he wants to show is that to acknowledge our ignorance, which is the scientist's starting point, is the first step to its cure. Only a human being knows how ignorant he is. Animals never do. This is why we learn more and lift ourselves up out of a merely instinctual existence into a cultural life.

A backlash can take either of two forms—disappointment when a promise is not fulfilled or a fear that it *will* be fulfilled. Sir Frank MacFarlane Burnet, the distinguished Australian, has said that work like Lederberg's in genetics may be "an evil thing." Admitting that he, Burnet, is a "temperamental pessimist," he felt that "there are dangers in knowing what should not be known."[25] This mood of a self-confessed pessimist is representative of a certain bloc in all walks of life, at all levels. Burnet will not agree that all knowledge is good, or that while there may be bad scientists there is no bad science.

The no-no and go-go postures have confronted each other on every frontier, including the biological, beginning with the discovery of fire. Over against Burnet's stance is the opinion of Elizabeth Boggs, past president of the National Association for Retarded Children: "I enter strong dissent to the proposition that we interpose any legal barriers or moral sanctions against any sober research, simply on the ground that we do not want anyone to know what might be discovered."[26]

An editorial writer in the American Medical Association, characteristically, has urged delaying tactics in the case of fertilized egg implants—apparently in the belief that a go-later policy is a third option and somehow different from no-no. In an editorial in its *Journal* he said, "The time seems clearly at hand to declare a moratorium on experiments that would attempt to implant an *in vitro* conception into a woman's womb."[27]

This may be only a hesitation waltz, a temporizing position motivated by medical politics. A somewhat more qualified proposal is that experiments on primates be fully carried out first, in the hope that monkeys are near enough like humans to establish whether the procedure is desirable for women patients and for the embryos thus conceived.[28]

Conflicts of this kind are not merely abstract or academic. Argument has promptly crystallized around Senator Mondale's proposal, supported by many other senators, for a National Advisory Commission on the Health Sciences and Society (Senate Joint Resolution 75).** It would bring lawyers, doctors, biologists, philosophers, sociologists, and theologians together to discuss the ethical and legal merits and probable social consequences of recent biological innovations. It could help to qualify the sheerly laissez-faire policy now in force. The Commission would make no prejudgments nor ask for controls. It would exist for only two years and make a report of its findings and recommendations.

A parallel proposal is for an international commission of the same kind.[29] A United Nations group, the Council for International Organizations of Medical Science, made the proposal in Paris in 1972. Unfortunately, the more vocal of its moving spirits are vigorous opponents of some or all of the new birth technologies, and it is believed by officials of the Council that UNESCO and WHO will not support it because of the potentially controversial debates.

If war is too important to be left solely up to the generals then biology is too important to be left to the biologists alone. Yet at once cries of protest arose against Senator Mondale's proposal. There is considerable scientific and medical opposition, based on a not unreasonable fear of ignorant or hasty interference from the know-nothing agitators. Some of the latter

** Its proposals have since been incorporated in H.R. 7724, favorably reported out of a committee chaired by Senator Edward Kennedy. This new bill converts the Commission into a permanent one with regulatory powers. Its aim is directly at clinical research only but obviously that means it would affect all biomedical development indirectly. Scientific and Congressional opinion is therefore divided as to its desirability.

have said that there is really nothing to be investigated anyway because all such "tinkering with human beings" is wrong. In fact, there would probably be both no-no and go-go viewpoints represented on the Commission—and there certainly should be.

The no-no forces will want to use the Commission to crack down with police powers in an attempt to purge scientific literature of the *verboten* subjects and, presumably, make foreign publications contraband. For example, the proposal just mentioned to hold up *in vitro* fertilizations and implants until primate tests are finished was accompanied by a call for "sanctions" on those who do not comply, by expelling them from scientific societies and denying them funds for research. No-noers do not seem to understand that the repression they advocate is precisely the kind of dictatorship they are afraid would be brought into being by the knowledge they are trying to repress.

As Lederberg puts it on behalf of free scientific investigation in general, "We have already experienced the sad consequences of the confusion of law with private morals in such areas as contraception and abortion and have only begun to extricate ourselves from the attendant hypocrisy and class discrimination."[30]

On the other hand, the go-go forces will have to stand up and answer serious questions about the uses their research should and should not be put to. Repressive reaction and uncritical demands for novelty are the Scylla and Charybdis between which we will have to chart a course to keep off the rocks.

This great debate will certainly run into a lot of mere noise and heat for a while, before we begin to see light. Deep-seated sentiments are at stake; learning or relearning is painful when it is genuine. Already the use of word weapons, language knives, is at work in the form of inflammatory adjectives and nouns. Lederberg has deplored the emotional effects sought by those who speak of "genocide" and "genetic tampering" when genetic therapy is discussed. He says it is like saying that education is "thought control" and calling the policy of making English the official language "cultural genocide."[31]

There is also dishonesty. One pronatalist author who will remain unnamed quoted George and Muriel Beadle's *The Language of Life* as saying we have "an inalienable right . . . to bear children" when in fact the Beadles had said that society, to counter overpopulation and genetic defects, may well have to limit any such claim to reproduce without interference.[32]

Of course, no experienced builder or planner can go ahead shutting his eyes to the remote as well as the immediate consequences of his efforts. It is foolish to eat mince pie if you have a disordered colon; the instant pleasure is not worth a night of lost sleep. Serious questions—problematic and not easily weighed— are raised, for example, about the dysgenic effect of *not* controlling the quality of the babies we bring into the world. Our biological mastery of life has certain unwelcome side effects when we fail to guard against them. One is the population explosion.

A second side effect is longevity. In 1900, in the United States a baby had forty-seven years of life coming to it on the average. In 1930, the prospect was for fifty-four years. In 1967, it had become seventy and a half years, chiefly due to improvements in the past seventy-five years in sanitation, nutrition, and preventive medicine. Life expectancy for people who refuse medical care, for example, Christian Scientists, is only about a year less than the average, which shows that after all it is not medical care but preventive health systems which have done the job of extending the life span.[33] But however the added years have come they are a big contributory factor in our population explosion.

A third and ominous side effect of the new sophisticated medicine is that it can spread genetic weaknesses and deformities. The number of mongoloids†† has been tripled or quadrupled because of improved neonatal (newborn) surgery and support systems. Until recently many of these pathetic creatures died quickly of untreatable complications like stomach blockages or imperforate anuses.[34] Ingenious remedies for pyloric stenosis, for example, a genetic or inborn disorder, which blocks the stomach from the intestine, spreads the gene for it by saving the afflicted so that they can pass it on in their progeny. It is increasing at something like 10 per cent from generation to generation—from 5 in 1,000 boys to 5.5 in the next generation, 6 in the next, and so on. The rate of occurrence in girls is only one fifth as high, but it spreads just as fast. There are many other ways by which *medicine* is polluting our common gene pool.

Could we, should we, have the heart to outlaw glasses and insulin because they help astigmatics and diabetics to survive and breed? It is only a step up the ladder of genetic therapy from these things to the more expensive and time-absorbing practice of giving dietary treatment to PKU babies. At what point does it become counterproductive? Where do we stop? For example, a Tay-Sachs enzyme assay, a simple blood test for all Ashkenazi Jews in the United States, would, it is estimated, cost only one fifth to one third what their defective children born in ignorance cost—in money, frustration, and heartache.

†† This name for mental deficiency is a gratuitous insult to the people of Mongolia, and we should call it Down's syndrome or 21-trisomy (because of the extra or forty-seventh chromosome which is its cause). "Trisomic" is the word, not Mongolian.

By what cost-benefit analysis can we decide such questions? How much are we willing to pay for the survival of genetically defective individuals—the payment measured in terms of the suffering of the "saved" ones, the burden on the family, and the economic drain on society? Here is an unwelcome new problem of social ethics foisted on us by the new biology.

Each of us has a genetic "load" of three to eight defects. This could double in two hundred years if we go on spreading genetic disorders through random sexual reproduction, multiplying the illnesses and costs that result from bad genes. This increase used to be offset by death and natural selection, but now the weak are preserved and protected. Which is better, to give up sanitation and medicine and social security, or give up random reproduction? We might survive as a society with a doubled load of bad genes, but think of the enormous cost in medicine, surgery, artificial aids, and diet controls for the increased numbers of victims. Life would lose its zest biologically as illness spread, and it would cease to be just a joke when inquiries about a patient's health were answered, "I'm afraid I'm going to live."

As one great geneticist, Theodosius Dobzhansky, sees it, the problem is that if "we enable the weak and the deformed to live and to propagate their kind, we face the prospect of genetic twilight; but if we let them die or suffer when we can save or help them, we face the certainty of a moral twilight."[35] He then concludes, "Each genetic condition will have to be considered on its own merits . . ." That is the clinical approach, each case taken on its own ground. It expresses the true spirit of medicine as well as situation ethics. Terrible and uncorrectable fetuses will have to be aborted or, after birth, let go; for those that *are* preserved and are able to live to reproductive maturity sterilization can prevent the spread of the bad genes and obviate the dysgenic side effect.

Choosing Between Right and Wrong

The proposal to consider each case on its own merits faces us with the question: How are we to tackle problems of right and wrong or of good and evil. This is perhaps the most radical ethical issue, the one that goes to the roots of morality. Is a human act right or wrong in and of itself, intrinsically, or is it right or wrong only extrinsically, according to the circumstances? Is it always wrong, for example, to lie or to steal or to fornicate?

Situation ethics says that the variables in any case determine what we ought to do, so that what is right sometimes is wrong other times, and this would be because the circumstances in one case would make an action (let's say abortion or sterilization) the right or best thing to do, even though in other cases the same action would be wrong because it would not contribute to the well-being of the people involved—their health, survival, growth, joy, social interest, self-realization, and so on.

The alternative to this is rule ethics, the belief that some things are inherently wrong whatever the mitigating circumstances might be. On this view some things are absolutely and always right or wrong, i.e., they are "universalized." Sometimes, however, the champions of rule ethics are compassionate and willing to justify or excuse an "intrinsically evil" deed because the rule conflicts with human need in a particular situation. But be it noted that this leavening or permissiveness is nothing more than that; it says only that although the action classified as wrong can be excused in such cases it is nevertheless still *wrong*.

Late in 1972, at a regional conference of the Florence Crittenden Association of America, which has for a long time been mobilizing help for unwed mothers, their officials announced a belated plan to open a Boston clinic for abortions. One of them said apologetically, "To many of us, abortion is a new and distasteful concept. To some it is intolerable." But her plea was that the need is very great and they therefore ought to provide abortions "if, after careful counseling, it proves wisest for that particular individual."

The basic ethical issue is whether abortion, if it is the "wisest" thing to do, is an evil act which can be excused—or, on the other hand, is a positively good thing to do. In this book it will be held that if any act or policy is the wisest as measured by human need and well-being, then it is *positively* good, *positively* the right thing to do. There will be no reason to have to defend it by some twisty kind of casuistry. This holds whether it is abortion, sterilization, artificial insemination, embryo implants, cloning, or any of the other matters we will discuss. What it comes down to is the conclusion that it is silly to say in any situation, however infrequently it occurs, that the right thing to do is wrong.

Dr. Dobzhansky's solution, to take each case on its own merits, sooner or later runs into the so-called "wedge argument" or entering wedge or slippery slope argument. May we ever do things which as a class carry the possibility of misuse or abuse? The heart of the "slippery slope" contention is that if you do anything which has or may have evil effects, even though you do it only for the sake of its good results, and even if the good outweighs the evil, you will tend more and more to tolerate the evil involved, until you stop caring. Therefore you ought never to do it all.

This amounts to an arbitrary refusal to risk "the thin edge of the wedge." The relative weight of the good gained would be of no avail in the wedge argument, not even when the evil entailed is clearly outweighed. Sometimes this ploy is called the camel's-nose-under-the-tent argument. In any case it comes down, as Paul Freund of the Harvard Law School has pointed out in a quotation from F. M. Cornford, to the view that nothing should be done for the first time.[36]

It is only a "so-called" argument because obviously its basis lies in a mood rather than rationally in logic, and its employers rely on what logicians call a "parade of horrors" for its effect. It consists of a deductive syllogism pretending to be inductive reasoning; actually it is merely hypothetical.‡‡ It runs this way: Major premise—exceptions from a general principle would result in the end of the principle; Minor premise—marital-sexual reproduction is an important principle; *Ergo*—cloning or artificial insemination and enovulation or genetic designing or artificial modes of baby making as such are wrong because they would destroy marriage and sexual reproduction. (We shall see more of this techniphobia in the chapters to follow.)

In another issue it takes the form, "If you use your powers to control quality by terminating a pregnancy in some prenatal cases, even though there is a severe disorder, you will get used to doing it and terminate even those with only minor defects—say a brachy-

---

‡‡ It has been used to justify the prohibition of alcohol and marijuana, divorce, anesthesia, public education, birth control, euthanasia, income taxes, almost any innovation you can name. It simply wipes out moral questions about drawing a line between constructive and destructive actions by taking refuge in a universal negative.

dactyl or short-fingered fetus; you will begin doing it with microcephalic newborns, but go on from that to terminate because of harelips."

This is a psychological block, not logical reasoning. As a prediction it is, at least for most sophisticated people, too simplistic and unqualified to make good sense. Surgeons do not refuse to "maim" a victim of gangrene because they might start amputating legs with poison ivy on them. Governments do not hesitate to arm their citizens in the national defense for fear the soldiers will go kill crazy—even though *some* will. (More of them are apt to turn pacifist.)

The greater good or lesser evil is a daily choice we have to make. For example, it *could* be (nobody believes it) that a method of uterine diagnosis called amniocentesis might lower the I.Q. potential of a fetus by say 10 to 15 points. This might not be shown to be true until a decade from now, for which reason it is important to keep a central registry of cases. But it would be foolish to stop doing amniocenteses because of the possibility, and it might still be defended because of the good it does even if it were true.

We should note, indeed, that the wedge objection *cuts both ways:* If we refuse to do a thing which bears the possibility of abuse for fear we will find it easier and easier to tolerate the evil, then we will by the same token find it easier and easier to tolerate the loss of the good. If we will not pay a price or run a risk for the sake of making quality children we will soon be indifferent to their miseries and lack of quality.

Hidden in this objection is a contempt for ordinary human beings, a belief that people have little or no value perception or capacity to discriminate. The philosopher Marvin Kohl declares, "It is important to strike out against the view which maintains that new or heterodox views of morality ought not to be considered or taught, because the masses are unintelligent. Although this is a favorite elitist tactic, it is, nonetheless, pernicious nonsense."[37]

Actually this obstructionist device, the wedge argument, has no place in standard works on philosophical ethics or moral theology. Yet it surfaces from time to time in the more conservative writers. Indeed, it is the quintessence of conservatism. The classical moralists' reply to it historically has been *abusus non tollit usum*, the abuse of a thing does not bar its use. The temper back of such a no-no position is not to be confused with the virtue of prudence. Prudence takes calculated risks in a trade-off spirit. It acts pragmatically for the sake of a proportionate good and does not flatly rule out all risks of undesired consequences regardless of the amount of good at stake.

Those who resort to such devices as the "wedge" are of course arguing on the ground of alleged consequences. On other questions or in other places they sometimes repudiate "consequential" reasoning in favor of an appeal *a priori* to the "inherent immorality" of biological innovations such as artificial inseminations and laboratory fertilizations.[38]

Trying To Be Natural

The uneasiness behind lots of opposition to biological control is related often to a feeling that the natural is better than the artificial. This is true enough sometimes but when it is it will be because of the particular situation. The natural is not intrinsically superior to the artificial. Medicine, for example, "interferes" with nature's business; it "manipulates" natural forces and tries to save our lives when nature left alone would finish us off with disease or deformity. Infant mortality is a natural process; so is pernicious anemia.

Art, artifice, the artificial—these are creative manipulations of what we find "raw" in nature, from the sculptor's marble to the surgeon's bone and flesh. For example, the chemical contraceptive "pill" brings about a simulated or pseudo pregnancy—as far as the biological system goes. It suspends ovulation, as pregnancy does. Nowadays more women at any one time are falsely pregnant than actually. But just because this is unnatural it is not antinatural or nonnatural. The unnatural is simply our control over the blind workings in raw natural processes. (The only antonym for natural is "supernatural"—a religious idea, incidentally, which is by no means accepted by all religious believers.)

Whatever can happen, with or without intelligent control, is natural. Natural does not mean merely the usual or typical. We can say, indeed, that whatever is, is natural. The word natural, like God, creation, and soul, is a "panchreston"—it explains everything in general and nothing in particular. Man is "higher" than the lower animal orders because of his intelligence, his brain capacity—those precious layers of cerebral cortex. It is precisely artificiality which is man's hallmark. Dr. Willard Gaylin of the Columbia University College of Physicians and Surgeons points out that men are characterized by techniques and that those who downgrade technology are engaging in "self-hatred."[39]

Innovations like genetic control have always been resisted by those who fear the built-in potential for misuse, which is a part of almost everything. It has been true of radio, TV, printing, automobiles, airplanes. Of such things we can and must always say that we hope control will work and we *know* that suppression will not work.

Speaking of social rather than biological controls Karl Marx in a famous marginal note expressed the essence of revolution: "The philosophers have only interpreted the world . . . the point is to change it." So we might say of genetics and the new birth technologies. The midwifery stage of birth and baby making in the past only tried to understand reproduction, but modern medicine is changing it. The jump from "taking what you get" by way of random or lottery conceptions to selective genetic and fetal engineering is a big jump indeed. But further than that, postmidwifery obstetrics is still entirely natural and being artificial is supremely human—humanely motivated and humanly manipulated.

Our basic ethical choice as we consider man's new control over himself, over his body and his mind as well as over his society and environment, is still what it was when primitive men holed up in caves and made fires. Chance versus control. Should we leave the fruits of human reproduction to take shape at random, keeping our children dependent on the accidents of romance and genetic endowment, of sexual lottery or what one physician calls "the meiotic roulette of his parents' chromosomes"?[40] Or should we be responsible about it, that is, exercise our rational and human choice, no longer submissively trusting to the blind worship of raw nature?

It is depressing, not comforting, to realize that most people are accidents. Their conception was at best unintended, at worst unwanted. There are those who are so bemused and befuddled by a fatalist mystique about nature with a capital N (or "God's will") that they want us to accept passively whatever comes along. Talk of "not tinkering" and "not playing God" and snide references to "artificial" and "technological" policies is a vote against both humanness and humaneness. The biologist George Gaylord Simpson once remarked that just as guinea pigs are not pigs nor from Guinea so "natural law" is neither law nor natural.[41]

Socrates thought it better to be an unhappy man than a happy pig. The pig's satisfaction with things as they are contrasts with a human being's struggle to make things better. Willingness to run the risks of requisite change and improvement is what makes human beings human. Humanness is courage married to reason. Pascal said (*Pensées*, 347) that man may be only a reed but he is a *thinking* reed; "our whole dignity consists in thought." Hence, man takes the tiller ethically. For Pascal adds, "By thought we must raise ourselves, not by space and time, which we cannot fill. Let us strive then to think well—therein is the principle of morality."[42]

Our birth strategies are basically of three kinds: (1) *eugenic*—this kind works without making any change in existing genes or fetuses and newborns, depending for its success on selective mating and selective abortion; (2) *euphenic*—this is a designed modification and control of either genetic defects or congenital anomalies, whether they are found in the fetus while still in the womb or not discovered until after birth. Modern fetology with its surgical penetration of the uterus to save Rh anemia fetuses would be an instance, or using a special diet to correct for a newborn's PKU (phenylketonuria), a genetic disease. Only the consequences of the genes are treated, not the DNA molecules and chromosomes themselves; (3) *genetic*—here we have the most fundamental strategy of all for the prevention of birth faults. It is a procedure to change the genes themselves, and their combinations, the basic building blocks of human beings, by deliberately directed mutations—rather than having to wait or hope for "spontaneous" mutants to just happen along.

As we shall see, genetic engineering is the thorniest area ethically because it is biologically the least worked out but the most elemental. H. J. Muller, the Indiana geneticist, once remarked that "we have about as much to be ashamed of in ourselves genetically as to be proud of," and that is probably the kernel fact.[43] Heredity plays a part in more than fifteen hundred diseases, and many of us are carrying time bombs— just waiting to explode with the right sexual combination, and as time goes along the chances are greater and greater.

To "get with it" in this new world we will have to stop talking foolishness; for example, talking about good and bad blood lines. What counts is genes, not corpuscles. People are very helpless as things stand; they know far more about their cars than they do about themselves.

II

SOME FACTS

Taking a hard look at what is right or wrong in modern reproduction, as well as at our efforts to exert quality control over it, we ought to start first with the state of the art—what the facts are—before we tackle any moral issues. On the new biological front the uninformed are more a part of the problem than of its solution. Sheer ignorance is as ominous as misinformation. The picture drawn in what follows has taken shape so quickly and so recently that some of us may not find it credible.

Genetic engineering as defined by the American Medical Association "might be considered as covering anything having to do with the manipulation of the gametes or the fetus, for whatever purpose, from conception other than by sexual union, to treatment of disease in utero, to the ultimate manufacture of a human being to exact specifications."[1] Although the "biological manufacture of human beings to desired specifications" is still a long way ahead of us, it is already very much a part of the ethics of reproduction.

By 1972, we knew of *eight* different ways to make babies. Most are accomplished facts and the others are just around the corner—close enough at hand to be treated as real, actual problems in morality. This was not true even in our own parents' time, a quarter century ago. There is indeed a generation gap.

The base line for this complex pattern of reproduction is still the age-old mode of coital intercourse followed by conception and the embryo's development (gestation) in the womb, ending in birth. This is what is historically familiar to us, the modality we had once supposed to be fixed and permanent—as fixed as lung breathing has been since we crawled up out of the sea onto the land. But this physiological mode of baby making can now at least be backed up by alternatives. Sex and family problems are consequently different now, and this is why we are having to take stock of both the facts and the questions raised by the facts.

The eight modes or methods of parenting can be listed very simply.[2] (1) The coital-gestational way. (2) Artificial insemination of a wife with her husband's sperm, without any assistance or input from a third party. (3) Artificial insemination of a woman with a donor's sperm. (4) Egg transfer* from a wife, inseminated by her husband and then transferred to another woman's womb for substitute gestation. (5) Egg transfer from a donor to a wife or unmarried woman's womb, before or after insemination—sometimes called prenatal adoption. (6) Egg transfer from a female donor, then inseminated by a male donor, and finally transferred to the recipient's womb. (7) Artificial gestation or nurture of a fetus in a glass womb or similar artifact—which is just a refinement of the incubator and isolette already in use for pre-

---

* Transfer is the right word, not transplant. This is because there is no tissue conjunction of the kind that takes place in skin or organ transplants which grow directly into the recipient's flesh. Transferred ova are implanted but they are not planted into the hostess' body. The egg is contained in her womb and nurtured in the placenta without being a part of *her*. (Actually, an embryo is a parasite and depends upon the woman's body but is not a part of her.) If it was a true transplant the immunity reaction would reject it, which is what happens in organ transplants with discouraging frequency.

mature infant—plus an artificial placenta; this is often spoken of as ectogenesis. (8) Nuclear transplant or cloning, whereby an egg (one's own or another's) is enucleated or denucleated; the original nucleus with its genetic code is removed and replaced with the nucleus of either a donated unfertilized egg or the nucleus from a body cell (either a man's or a woman's), which is then implanted and brought to term in one's own or another's womb—and all this *without conception*. Only a male or a female seed is used, not both. It is birth from only one parent, *artificial* virgin birth.

Looking at Alternatives

Looked at biologically we might say that there are really only *five* truly different modes: coitus and then gestation by one woman, artificial insemination, egg transfer, artificial gestation, and nuclear transplant. Only the first mode, coitus-gestation, is nontechnical. All the others are biotechnical—forms of rational artificial assistance to human reproduction in one manner or degree or another.

The first seven of the first, longer, list are different modes of sexual reproduction. All are effected through conception or fertilization, i.e., by the union of both male and female sex cells either in a Fallopian tube or a test tube. Only the last one on the list, the nuclear transplant, is asexual—without conception or fertilization. To use the biologists' language, they are "replications from a single cell" rather than from a pair of germ cells or "gametes" sexually combined.

There is still another method, a potential ninth one, which as yet is only a "far out" or speculative option for humans. It is known as monogenesis. In raw nature the process is one of spontaneous embryo development from one gamete or sex cell only, an egg or a sperm, not the normal combination of the two. An embryo can develop not only in diploid fashion, when two sex cells and their chromosomes combine—the usual thing—but also in haploid fashion. This means that only one germ or sex cell's chromosomes participate. They are precipitated into the growth process either spontaneously or by being induced.

This can be done chemically, electrically, or mechanically. Rabbits' eggs can be started off by cooling them; frogs' eggs, by a pinprick through the membrane. In nature the sperm sometimes activates the egg but fails to fuse with its nucleus; in this case the embryo has only female chromosomes and it is called gynogenesis. Sometimes (less frequently) the egg's nucleus fails to enter into combination, leaving only male chromosomes, and this is called androgenesis. Creatures born of either gynogenesis or androgenesis are motherless, not in the sense of having lost her but of never having had one.

This kind of reproduction therefore is asexual, just as cloning is. However, although the individual produced is necessarily of the same sex as its mono-parent it will by no means be identical, either in physique or in personality. Monogenesis is sometimes called parthenogenesis, or *virgin* birth. In nature it occurs chiefly in plants and invertebrate animals, but it may happen naturally or be induced in frogs, bag moths, rabbits, and even some turkeys. Its occurrence among humans is estimated at anywhere from zero to about once in 1.6 million pregnancies. (Cloning in fact is artificial parthenogenesis, or technological virgin birth.)

If monogenesis were ever to become a part of human birth technology it would be a far simpler modality than cloning. No intricate renucleation of an ovum is needed—no nuclear transplant is involved. But although it is a possibility and far more than mere science fiction, it still lies on the far edge of workability.

In what follows we will restrict our discussion to the first eight modes, leaving monogenesis to the day, near or distant, when it reaches a more practical status.†

What all this adds up to is that we have moved from contraceptive or quantity control to a sophisticated reproductive medicine aiming at *quality* birth control. The family-planning slogan "Stop the Stork" is misleading. The problem is to control the stork, not to stop it. And to share parenthood around more evenly. There are in the neighborhood of 2,500,000 childless couples in this country who could be helped by these new birth technologies to outwit the frustrating indifference of raw nature.

Conception no longer depends on coital intercourse *in vivo*. Now it can take place artificially, *in vitro*. Literally this means "in glass," but as a laboratory procedure it refers to putting the egg and sperm together artificially in any container, with a liquid solution of appropriate nutrients. The artificially fertilized conceptus may then be implanted in the uterus of a human body and brought to term, as in egg transfers. With the glass womb they will be gestated as well as fertilized *in vitro*.

We have a considerable variety of combinations and permutations in reproductive methods. All but the

.† In some sense we might say that hybridization and cell-tissue fusion is still another mode. Man-animal "hybrids," modern Gorgons and Minotaurs are being investigated. Work goes forward also on man-machine "hybrids" or cyborgs, combining human bodies and mechanical-electric adjuncts. But we are dealing only with the morality of human reproduction, not with postnatal innovations and manipulations.

last two of the eight in our list are actually in practice or actually practicable. Nuclear transplants (clonings) for humans are thought to be within ten years of realization; already they are being done in simpler creatures like carrots and frogs. Artificially duplicating the placenta holds up artificial gestation but a sudden breakthrough in biochemistry could put it within the reach of clinical practice—just as a faster advance in cytology (cell research) could jump nuclear transplants ahead even faster than we have supposed.

What we must keep in mind is that all of these things are perfectly natural. They are all based on biology, on the life sciences. Technology is after all nothing but a combination of human reason and natural processes which reinforces, alters or replaces "nature's" way of doing things.‡ But technology cannot be "against nature" because in that case it simply could not work. These artificial modes of baby making or parenting may seem strange or even bizarre, but if asexual reproduction seems bizarre to our minds, accustomed as we are to sexual methods, sexual reproduction could seem bizarre to other species.

These different modes of controlled human baby making also involve a growing list of techniques still more or less unfamiliar to most people. The list includes sterilization permanently or temporarily; the biochemistry of infertility treatment—for example, hormone therapy or such devices as correcting oligospermatic semen (too few sperm) by mixing several

‡ An ethical distinction is made in Catholic moral theology. Anything is wrong if it undermines or prevents "an end intended by nature," they say, e.g., contraception or abortion or sterilization, but whatever *assists* "an end intended by nature" is permissible—e.g., contact lenses or a cane or an implanted heart pacemaker. All of these new technical modes of reproduction aid a natural process, they do not hinder. Moral objections will therefore have to rest on other grounds, as we shall see.

ejaculates and inseminating artificially; embryatrics or fetal surgery and medicine; amniocentesis; pregnancy termination; cold storage of sperm and eggs (cryobanking); gonad grafts; placental research; hybridization or tissue-fusion technology; prenatal sex or gender selection; and molecular biology—genetics, virology, cytology, and enzyme use.

In a speculative way we can also foresee new methods of radical transsexualization. Surgical conversion of genitalia is already in practice for people who feel themselves to be of the other sex and who may even have been born hermaphroditic or intersexual anatomically. (Note that this is not homosexuality, which is sex relations between persons of the same gender. On the contrary, it is a physical conversion for the sake of heterosexual relations.)

Furthermore, transplant or replacement medicine foresees the day, after the automatic rejection of alien tissue is overcome, when a uterus can be implanted in a human male's body—his abdomen has spaces—and gestation started by artificial fertilization and egg transfer. Hypogonadism could be used to stimulate milk from the man's rudimentary breasts—men too have mammary glands. If surgery could not construct a cervical canal the delivery could be effected by a Caesarean section and the male or transsexualized mother could nurse his own baby.

In this way we would see the realization of what were thought to be old wives' tales in China about men wet-nursing infants. As it is at present, women have four reproductive functions: to menstruate, ovulate, gestate, and lactate—while men only impregnate. But euphenic and genetic surgery may soon be trading these functions back and forth; they have already begun doing it with both surgery and hormones.

Stages Along Life's Way

Control over baby making operates at three levels: the *contraconceptive*, the *prenatal*, and the *preconceptive*. On the first two levels we are well launched, and the preconceptive—controlling the basic genetic makeup of a new individual—is not as far behind as some may think. Fetology reaches back through the birth barrier to treat embryonic life in the womb, and genetics reaches back through the conception barrier to control the primal stuff that enters into the origin of human lives.

We are all familiar with artificial conception preventers—the pill and sheath, the intrauterine device (IUD), cervical caps, foams, douches. Recent work in pharmacology is close to perfecting night-before and morning-after pills, releasing women from the elaborate burden of the steroids now in use. We may expect the advent any time of implantable time-release capsules, suspending ovulation for as much as a year per capsule.

Truculent women's liberation advocates have accused medical people of male chauvinism because the onus of most contraceptive controls has fallen thus far to the female. But this is the case only because the female's biological system offers many more points of control than the male's. The search for male "oral pills" has met with little success as yet. Biochemistry is looking for a way to suspend the "capacitation" of sperm and already a diamine is known which is not toxic but stops sperm production temporarily. (It also creates an intolerance to alcohol, thus killing two birds with one stone—unwanted pregnancies and addictive drinking.)

No method of contraception, however, is as simple and safe as sterilization. As early as 1970, 16.3 per cent of couples in this country had been sterilized (as against 34.2 per cent, only twice as many, using the pill).[3] Sterilization will advance, "contraception" will decline. Male ligations or vasectomies totaled 750,000 in 1970; an estimated 3,000,000 men have had it done—a simple office procedure of a few minutes. Feminine sterilization by laparascope, a lens and electrocoagulating instrument inserted through the abdomen, known as band-aid or belly-button surgery, takes only a couple of hours all told. It is legal now in all fifty states.

The pill itself is really a sterilizer, temporarily suspending ovulation. Since its use is complicated and unfairly onerous for the woman, it will be superseded when a good reversible surgical sterilization is perfected, perhaps by a removable metal or plastic microvalve or plug for male and female tubes. In any case, neither contraception nor sterilization is *birth* control; they are conception control. Abortion is the only birth control—if we use our language carefully. Chemical abortifacients (abortion-causing drugs) such as the "morning-after pill" and others which may be soon developed from the so-called prostaglandins** and mechanical safeguards such as the intrauterine device are overlaps of both contraception and abortion. Since they do not prevent conception, however, they are really abortive measures.

Some international medical groups have suggested that conception should be understood to take place only when the blastocyst has reached the uterus and implanted itself in the endometrium, the lining of the womb. This would mean that conception takes place

** Only so-called because they are misnamed. This group of biochemical agents comes from semen, not as first believed from the prostate gland.

not at fertilization but several days later. Given this definition the term "conceptus" for tubal plasma or fertilized ova prior to implantation would have to be dropped. It would also mean that those who claim a conceptus is a human person from fertilization onward are claiming not that conception but *fertilization* is the start of a person.††

Contraception and sterilization only control quantity; *quality* control is achieved by a combination of the new fetal medicine with selective abortion. By definition abortion on demand or at request could be for reasons other than medical, yet in its own way it too might be said to be a method of quality control, just as contraception and sterilization are.

Prenatal control, consisting of fetal therapy backstopped by abortion, is a striking example of this two-sidedness. At the prenatal level of reproductive medicine, compared to the contraconceptive, the aim is to *achieve* new life, not to prevent it. But when obstetrical care is concerned about the quality of new life, not willing to passively just accept any kind of baby that happens to come along, *caring* may entail abortion when an embryo or fetus is found to be both seriously and incurably defective.

This is why physicians in genetic counseling usually make sure in advance that when parents want to know what the prospects are for a fetus *in utero* they will be willing to have it terminated if the prenatal diagnosis is "positive"—i.e., if the evidence reveals some

†† This would apply to the traditional Catholic doctrine that a "human being" exists prior to implantation. For those who pinpoint conception at implantation, however, flushing fertilized ova from the tubes would not be immoral or a "malicious" ending of human life. But all of this is little more than word mongering. Loose language, which is much too widespread in these matters, is a sign of loose thinking.

serious genetic defect or congenital anomaly such as
Tay-Sachs disease (amaurotic idiocy) or Down's syndrome ("mongolism"). It would be cruel to make such
terrible diagnoses for worried parents if they believed,
for whatever reason, that they were morally obliged
to bring such a child into the world regardless of the
misery foreseeable for the baby and the family, to say
nothing of the interests of society at large. Yet parents should have the information if they want to know
what is ahead.

It is noteworthy from the standpoint of ethical concerns, according to Dr. John Littlefield of the Massachusetts General Hospital, that about one out of every
six couples who are told such bad news goes ahead
with the pregnancy anyway.[4] A study in England
showed that *two* out of six couples were undeterred
by the bad news.[5] On the other hand, in a report from
Johns Hopkins University in Baltimore, only one
couple in nine went on to conceive after being advised
of genetic or hereditary defects.[6]

As things stand now, such is the moral lag between
medical science and popular attitudes, there is no law
requiring genetically unfortunate people to give up
"normal" sexual reproduction and turn to adoption or
artificial insemination or egg transfer. Some doctors contend that bad gene carriers should be free to reproduce even when they know the truth, and that the
knowledge should be kept secret even from those persons such patients are planning to marry—if they elect
to deceive their affianced.[7] In a southern university
hospital recently a young man's hemophilia was reck-
oned to have cost his family, the hospital, and the
public pocket a total of one million dollars by the
time he decided to *marry and have children of his
own*.

In South Dakota a family cursed with an incurable dominant gene defect causing ataxia or spino-cerebellar degeneration, a progressive loss of speech and muscular control, has spread its disease like tumbleweed through dozens of families. It runs a course of fifteen to twenty years before death comes. Its onset comes in the late twenties, after marriage and children. It had been kept a "family secret" until 1970 when the facts were established by the National Institutes of Health, at the request of one family's doctor. NIH joined the conspiracy by giving its assurance that their test results would be kept secret in the files.

Only recently did the National Genetics Foundation in New York persuade these people to allow the facts to be published.[8] Some of them have had vasectomies but others have elected to take a 50-50 chance with having children. It is sometimes argued that a physician doing genetic counseling ought not as a physician to be motivated by broad social concerns, only by the therapeutic concern. Yet as one physician brought into the South Dakota case by the NGF puts it: "You could wipe out this disease within a generation, even without a cure, if the affected persons simply stop having babies."

A fetus is vulnerable to many kinds of ills. One kind of congenital defect would be when the Rh positive red blood cells of the fetus are destroyed by antibodies from the mother's Rh negative blood; other examples are damage from thalidomide in the early weeks of pregnancy, damage from radiation, and rubella. Such defects are injuries or infections occurring after conception, in the womb.

Other congenital ills might be genetic, either metabolic or chromosomal. They include recessive diseases such as phenylketonuria, a defect in the liver enzyme, and such dominant diseases as Huntington's chorea, which shows up only in the middle years of life; there are other things such as achondroplasia (dwarfism) and less serious maladies like myopia and diabetes. Inborn errors in metabolism (body chemistry) and faulty chromosomes in the original structure of the germ cells, the sperm and ova—these ills exist *before* conception. More than fifteen hundred genetic aberrations have been identified, and for over a hundred of them a specific enzyme deficiency has been traced to a gene source. The list is growing swiftly.

About 20 to 30 per cent of conceptuses, embryos and fetuses "die" by spontaneous (natural) abortion— a very high rate of loss. Almost all such aborts are defective, genetically or congenitally. Most abortions go unrecorded because they are not recognized for what they are; they are thought to be only unusually thick menstrual discharge. Spontaneous abortions and many miscarriages are a blessing. Nature takes the same way medicine does; it closes the book on failures.

Now that we know something about it we realize that contrary to popular sentiment the womb is a very dangerous place—a hazardous environment. The glass womb will offer a much safer and more easily monitored container for fetuses, a place where they can be more easily manipulated for treatment and salvation. Work on these incubators at Stanford University and elsewhere is held up for the present, in spite of the availability of the "hardware" to provide the chamber and oxygenation needed, because the key to providing an ex-uterine placenta has not been found yet by the biochemists. Without a proper artificial placenta to nullify the toxic effects of fetal urine and other wastes a fetus would soon arrest or "die" in an artificial womb.

Genetics the Real Frontier

The third level of reproductive medicine, the *pre-conceptive*, is the newest one and the most fundamental. As it opens up it reveals exciting possibilities of quality control for our children. Genetics is the true frontier now, with its discoveries about genes and the chromosomes. Chromosomes are the chains, or ladders, of genes which give us our physical traits. The "genotype" to a big extent, not totally, sets the "phenotype." For example, a Down's syndrome baby is mentally retarded, the victim of a mysteriously out-of-place forty-seventh chromosome—there should be only forty-six. The extra chromosome also causes an overdose of genes which results in multiple defects besides the mental one. This genetic disorder is now discoverable by fetal diagnosis. The next step will be to find some way to remove the offending chromosome. And so it will go with all the other genetic dangers.

Genetics has finally become medical. It is no longer just a study of the leaf curl in tobacco or ways which biochemists use to get mice to respond to insulin or why it is that Japanese get their hairy ear rims. Joshua Lederberg has coined the word "algeny" for it; just as the ancients tried to use alchemy to convert lead into gold, so molecular biologists seek ways to turn leaden inheritances into golden ones.

Genetic disorders are inherited in two ways. One kind are dominant gene diseases; they need to be present in only one parent but they affect both males and females and pass from generation to generation, with a 50-50 chance of reappearing in each child. The other kind are recessive; for the disease to show up in the child both of the parents must be carrying the gene recessively and then each child will stand on the average a 1-in-4 chance of inheriting the disease and a 50-50 chance of being a carrier—that is, one will have the disease, two will carry it, and one will be free of it. If only one parent is a carrier, half of the children will be carriers, half will be free of the harmful gene.

We all carry from three to eight lethal genes recessively—that is, they are "sleepers" lurking in the depths until we happen by chance to marry somebody who also carries the same bad gene. Then they unite and do their dreadful work. About 250,000 children are born every year with birth defects in this country and 20 per cent of them are due to known genetic causes. All of us has some genetic defect transmissible to our children.

They say that 10 per cent of sterile couples are sterile because of genetic defects and that 5 per cent of our children are lost because of genetic diseases before they reach maturity. These are family metabolic disorders like sickle cell anemia. Some are ruinous, some are tragic but sublethal, others are relatively minor— like gout (which can be very serious), obesity, and treatable diabetes. Some disorders if diagnosed prenatally or soon after birth can now be corrected. For example, a metabolic disease (meaning an enzyme defect in the body's chemistry) called galactosemia leads to cataracts and mental retardation, but if it is diagnosed at birth the effects can be prevented by keeping the milk sugar called galactose out of the child's diet for about three years.

It is estimated that about one fourth of our hospital beds are filled with victims of genetic disease, if we take into account the genetic factors in diseases like schizophrenia and diabetes.

The exciting thing about preconceptive medicine is that it promises us ways to prevent these genetic illnesses at the source, by fixing up the genes and chromosomal aberrations themselves—restructuring them at the alpha point, i.e., in their primary location, the cell. A great company of geneticists and cytologists (cell biologists), backed by biochemists and molecular biologists, is at work. Their teamwork is known as "cytogenetics."

The point about preconceptive medicine or "genetic engineering" in the narrow meaning of the term is that as it succeeds *it reduces the amount of human misery and cuts down the expensive and inconclusive struggle of postnatal medicine.* The latter can only come into play after the damage is done. It is important, furthermore, to note that *genetic engineering reduces the need to resort to abortion.*‡‡ Engineered changes in the cells become at once a part of the inheritance process, to be passed on through either sexual or asexual reproduction—except when spontaneous mutations might cancel them out.

A step in this direction is seen in the experimental fusion of cells, to introduce needed genes from healthy cells into defective or deficient ones. Viruses are used to carry genes in this procedure. For example, this has been claimed to supply a cell from a galactosemia sufferer with the missing gene, one which produces the enzyme needed to break down the galactose in milk. When the procedure achieves a permanent change in the cell, and when researchers learn how to find the right part of the patient's body to inject with the redeemed cell, so that its enzyme will spread to the other cells involved, a great feat of gene therapy will be complete.

‡‡ In a personal communication Joshua Lederberg says, "I am beginning to be skeptical about the practicability of this ideal. That is, for most diseases preemptive abortion is likely to be much more reliable than other therapy."

There are at least one hundred diseases due to a single bad gene, which therefore makes them good candidates for gene therapy. One such is Tay-Sachs disease, a fatal disorder of the nervous system mostly afflicting Jewish children; another disease is sickle cell anemia—a blood disorder which mainly shows up in black people. But when it comes to polygenic diseases like diabetes, due to a complex combination of *many* genes, the task is harder, as it is when the trouble lies not in genes as such, which would be the case in amaurotic idiocy, but in a whole extra chromosome—as in Down's syndrome.

Other strategies of gene therapy—as distinguished from genetic design—would be to implant normal cells (cells with the right genes and chromosomes) in developing embryos, or to synthesize viruses to carry the needed enzymes, called transduction. Enzymes and DNA (the genetic code of proteins that "instructs" our cells how to arrange themselves in bodily parts and functions) have been synthesized artificially and viruses have been artificially duplicated.

The extent to which gene therapy should be utilized is one about which biomedical experts are not agreed. Some have urged vigorous research and development, but at the same time want to hold up any actual practices until more is known of their long-term effects.[9] These procedures have actually been carried out already in bacterial and animal research. The purpose is literally to turn genes on and off at will. We can begin to appreciate the extent of the broad task of identifying and isolating gene functions for genetic control when we understand that there are literally hundreds of millions of nucleotide units in each set of chromosomes.

It has been found that a milligram of thyroxin from a fish or sheep will turn a gilled water newt into a land salamander. This is a small sample of what lies ahead in biochemistry as it pushes ahead.[10] Similar things have been done in insects with intranuclear grafting, a technique right on the threshold of managing interspecific hybrids (the merging of different species). At bottom genetics is chemistry.

The ultimate goal of genetic engineering is not to ameliorate the ills of patients prenatally or postnatally, but to start people off healthy and free of disease through the practice of medicine *preconceptively*. It is a matter of directed and rational mutations, over against the accidental mutations now going on blindly in nature. It aims to control people's initial genetic design and constitution—their genotypes—by gene surgery (transduction) and by genetic design (insertion and deletion). Besides biochemistry it might use micrometric or microscopic tools like laser light beams or anything else that serves the purpose.

When we recall how minute human germ cells are we can appreciate what a strange new world this is. A hen's egg shell can contain fifty thousand human ova, and one haploid human ovum contains (as does a sperm) twenty-three chromosomes, each chromosome with thousands of genes on it. Even so the naked eye can barely see a human egg and cannot see a human sperm at all. Yet genes are not merely trackable now; Dr. H. G. Khorana of the University of Michigan has artificially constructed a gene by organic chemistry, and Dr. James Danielli of Buffalo (State University of New York) has artificially synthesized a living cell. No wonder scientists talk about astronauts someday sowing Mars with artificially created forms of life, both vegetable and animal.

A certain gynecologist tells a story of feminine heroism that dramatizes the biological revolution, ranking along with anything told about Barbara Fritchie or Florence Nightingale. This physician checked a patient's pregnancy by amniocentesis, which means putting a thin cannula through the vaginal or abdominal wall into the amniotic sac, where the fetus nestles, to withdraw a sample of the fluid and study it for evidence of chromosomal aberrations. This is a method called karyotyping—a microscopic examination of the cell nuclei in the fluid. The test revealed a deadly defect, Tay-Sachs disease, in her fetus.

When she heard the bad news the patient decided to have the pregnancy terminated. The genetics were explained to her. An average of one in four fetuses conceived by her and her husband would have this, a mortal disease. The question was, should she be sterilized, her tubes tied off, and perhaps an adoption arranged? "No," she answered, "I will conceive again, and again and again if necessary, and I will abort and abort, until a sound and healthy child comes to us." That is what happened. Not until the fourth pregnancy did the disease fail to show up, and then a normal son was born to happy parents—responsible parents.

In another reported case, parents of a boy born with Duchenne muscular dystrophy decided not to have any more children, but after two years they heard of amniocentesis and elected to start another pregnancy and have it checked out. The test showed the fetus would be a girl, and girls are free of Duchenne. She was born altogether normal, but the wife explained that if it had been a boy fetus she would have had it terminated, as others have.

To cite another example of the need to test, a career woman who has postponed maternity ought to have tests for Down's syndrome. This is because at age twenty-five the chances of having a Down's baby are only one in twenty-five hundred but at forty-five the chances become one in fifty. Women over forty have only 2 per cent of all pregnancies, but they produce 22 per cent of the afflicted children.

Abortion has lost its terrors. A comparison of morbidity and mortality rates related to abortion and pregnancy shows a far higher incidence of trouble in pregnancy. *Abortion is far safer than pregnancy.* The growing practice of "menstrual extraction" in America and Europe, a method of clearing out the uterine lining with a suction syringe any time up to six weeks after the patient's period is missed, gets rid of the older technique of dilation and curettage (D & C) and can be done in a clinic or doctor's office in a few minutes. It is a physiologically negligible intervention, far simpler than any of the other new abortion methods— a "prophylactic abortion" before the usual pregnancy tests become reliable.

It is still true, everything else permitting, that the best time for an abortion is within the first trimester, medically regarded. However, the bad news of genetic or congenital trouble cannot be learned very early in pregnancy by present known means. An amniocentesis, for example, is not now practicable before twelve to fourteen weeks at the earliest, and so it is with various other uterine diagnoses and therapies. Even so, modern methods such as suction and hypertonic saline procedures, along with magnificent advances in obstetrical surgery, have enormously reduced the old-fashioned traumas and risks.

The Tactics of Quality Control

The three-prong combination of genetic counseling, prenatal care, and selective abortion of undesirable fetuses has become a splendid system of quality control. There are many psychological and ethical problems involved in the actual practice, some of which we shall be examining. The difference between "therapeutic abortion" in obstetrics and "selective abortion" in genetics is vague and unclear. Whatever it is called, however, abortion is an obvious remedy for unwanted pregnancies.

People who knowingly undertake or who only stumble into the conception of new life are learning that they may be carriers of serious genetic faults. If they have any sense of responsibility for quality in their offspring and of obligation to the community's interest they will want to know as much as they can about their inheritance, their gene pattern. They do not want, ignorantly and innocently, to pass on a bad dominant gene or join their germ cells with a partner's whose recessive bad gene matches their own, resulting in the victimization of their child and their own unhappiness.

Along with genetic diagnosis and counseling on a clinical or personal basis arises the policy problem of mass or social screening measures. About 90 per cent of people only turn to genetics after a defective baby is born; the rest do so because they happen to be worried about "something in the family inheritance."[11] Inherited disorders usually show up in children because the parents were unaware that they themselves carried the gene for a disease, or that one spouse did. Much of this kind of tragedy could be avoided if people had some genetic tests to show what their "sleepers" are, or a record of some kind to forewarn them. This would be private knowledge, for making personal or unilateral decisions on whether to marry and whether to reproduce.

But what about the partner? Should we have to rely on our mate's candor and concern? And what of society's stake in it? What if one or both of a pair of carriers chooses to disregard the facts? To meet these dangers proposals are being made to establish registers, the data to be fed in from findings of genetic counselors and ob-gyn services in clinics and hospitals. This, however, raises questions about privacy, scandal, who would have access to the information, the social interest and social control.*

There are two parts to the screening problem; the testing and the recording. Whether filed records should be kept comes down in the end to whether we think we can trust people to be truthful genetically. Linus Pauling, the Nobel prize winner, peace advocate, and Christopher Columbus of molecular biology (with his work on sickle cell anemia done in 1949) has suggested that carriers should wear a small tattoo on their foreheads as Indians wear caste marks. In many dominant gene defects the disease or deformity in its victims is obvious enough to plain sight. For example, Down's syndrome or amaurotic idiocy (after the first six months) or dwarfism. Recessive defects which remain unpaired or heterozygotic are unseen, but if both parents carry the same fault (are both heterozygotic) then it will show up because one fourth of their progeny are affected. If the gene is sex linked (for example, women are the carriers and men the victims in hemophilia) the moral question is the same. Chromosome defects consist of a whole package of genes, not just one—which is the case in some sterility problems, some mental retardates, some malformed people.

* In 1972 there were forty-three states which required hospital tests for PKU in all newborns. Some states, plus the District of Columbia, had compulsory screening laws for sickle cell anemia, but none required screening for Tay-Sachs—a fact which led to charges by blacks of discrimination. This black militant complaint makes some sense, but their charge that screening is genocide does not. Congress authorized $105 million for sickle cell prevention, but little was actually spent.

Apparently Pauling's suggestion is meant as a voluntary device only. Its aim is to keep recessive carriers from getting too fond of each other or—if they are already devoted—it would accustom them to the idea of artificial insemination (donor) or egg transfer (donor). Others believe that the social interest cannot rely upon the disinterestedness of people who carry recessive traits.

Mrs. Beeton's cookbook said of preparing jugged hare, "First catch your hare." In the same way, before we get to the question of how to handle information about genetic risks we have to get the information.

A few genetic diseases such as Tay-Sachs disease are more simply detected. In the Washington-Baltimore area in 1971 a voluntary mass screening program found 250 cases of carriers among 7,000 people tested; the estimate is that in the United States there are another 7,500 carriers not yet reached. In other major cities Jewish leadership is promoting similar screenings for Ashkenazi Jews. The test is a simple blood sampling. The real test of screening is in the success or failure of *voluntary* programs. A similar test, for sickle cell anemia among blacks, was carried out in District of Columbia schools. Carriers were found at the predictable rate (10 per cent), and the disease itself was actually present in the predictable proportion, 10 per cent of the children of carriers.

It is also possible to make skin-cell tests on fetuses, or to make them at delivery and even later. After all, genetic counseling tests and the tests proposed for marriage license examinations are often of this kind. Each and every one of our body or somatic cells, remember, contains all of our genetic information, the full genotype, from conception to death.

Prenatal care now includes many other monitoring devices. The fetus can be watched by microphones, electromicroscopes, infrared thermography, X ray, ultrasonics, radio-opaque dyes. Culdoscopy, a new method, is the insertion of a thin tube into the pelvic interior to take pictures (even motion pictures) of tubes, ovaries, uterus, and the whole reproductive system. Once we have the glass womb or placenta-lined incubator with a clear view of the contents it will be possible to monitor, diagnose, and treat problem fetuses. Many now being lost will be saved.

Fetal surgery will soon deal directly with lung hernias, hydrocephaly, tumors, and cardiovascular defects. And as we learn to fully diagnose fetal infections we may be able to inject requisite drugs to fight enemy parasites, bacteria, and viruses—for example, infectious hepatitis, polio, and rubella.

"Superfetation"—extra or multiple fetuses—will also be dealt with by fetal surgery. Superfetation results from superovulation; it is to be seen in the simultaneous fertilization of twins, triplets, quadruplets, quintuplets, sextuplets, etc. Dr. John Rock, a distinguished Catholic birth control pioneer at Harvard, began in the 1940s to do test-tube or *in vitro* fertilizations of the eggs from women patients. Since then scientists have learned how to stimulate or slow down an ovary's production of eggs and to extract the eggs, keeping them in nutrients, which are usually natural but may be artificially mixed fluids. This has proved to be an invaluable means to select the sex of children.

For some time there have been ways available to find out the sex of a fetus after a certain period of gestation. But now genetic studies of eggs and sperm *in vitro* (at the lab bench) have shown that human conceptuses carry a pair of chromosomes which show the sex of the individual. A male is XY, a female is XX. Eggs are always X but sperm may be either X or Y. Therefore, the sex of the conceptus is decided by whether the sperm that fertilizes the egg bears an X chromosome and produces a female or a Y chromosome and produces a male.

Using physical methods like centrifuge and electrophoresis, or chemical techniques such as chromatin color in female cells, experts can tell which is which. This means that they can induce superovulation in a patient and remove the eggs, which gives them many eggs to choose from for insemination *in vitro*. When they inseminate or fertilize them artificially they choose an XY (boy) or an XX (girl) conceptus, and implant or transfer it to a womb for nurture, discarding the surplus. This is a method already widely practiced in animal husbandry—as indeed nearly all of the seven artificial modes of reproduction are. Biology is biology, for one species as much as for another. Results to date are that about half of such implants are successful with animals, without abnormalities. "Teratologists" or specialists in factors causing distortion are busy investigating how animal methods may or may not be applied to human reproduction.

Several genetic diseases are linked to the sex chromosomes. Mention has been made of one, hemophilia. Another is muscular dystrophy, which kills the boy child but hangs on in the mother and sister to be passed on to more male victims unless sterilization or abortion prevent it. Also there are defects in the sex chromosomes themselves. For example, Klinefelter's syndrome is due to an extra X or female chromosome on the XY (male) code. This XXY results in effeminacy, retardation, behavior disturbances. An extra Y or male chromosome on the XY seems sometimes to lead to violence and criminal tendencies in such XYY men, although the effects of this particular karyotype are still in question. Extra chromosomes are definitely genetic causes of trouble, notably in the Down's syndrome—an extra one on the twenty-first rung of the cell's arrangement of chromosomes, which is why it is called "21-trisomy."

A normal ejaculate contains sperm of both X and Y kinds, gynosperms and androsperms. Ways are being considered to separate them, producing men who are gyno-fathers and men who are andro-fathers. If this works out women will be able to choose their partners in reproduction in order to determine a child's sex. A researcher at the National Institutes of Health has noted that male-making sperm are smaller than female-making sperm and proposes a vaginal diaphragm which lets only androsperm through. Some day would-be fathers may be taking pills before conception to regulate X or Y motility (pink pills for girls, blue for boys?). Sex selection will do a lot to stop "multiparity" or too many children, because "trying again" for a wanted boy or girl is a major cause of numerous pregnancies.

(Men can no longer put the blame on their wives when they get "all girls" or "all boys" now that we know it is the *man's* sperm that decides an embryo's sex. And with the new genetics hinterland farmers will have to give up hanging their overalls on the right-hand bedpost if they want a boy or the left-hand bedpost for a girl. There are more rational ways now to choose and control our children's gender.)

Human Germ Cell Sharing

Several years ago (1961) an Italian Catholic expert in interspecific or interspecies transplants (for example, putting calves' pituitary glands in human patients) got interested in the foreign tissue-rejection problem. How can we suppress the immunity reaction which rejects foreign tissue and brings so many brilliant transplant operations down in ultimate failure? In the course of his research Dr. Danielle Petrucci and his assistants reported that they had artificially fertilized a human embryo in the laboratory and had brought it forward through regular cell divisions (growth) for twenty-nine days. They saw then that it was teratogened (defective) and disposed of it.

Being uncertain whether his church would believe the embryo to be endowed with a soul or not he says he administered conditional baptism and extreme unction by a lay formula. His experiment was condemned as immoral by spokesmen for the church, because as a "test tube baby" it was artificial and because it involved abortion. (Embryologists speak of sacrificing or disposing of un-nidated or unimplanted embryos and of *aborting* nidated or implanted uterine tissue.) It seems strange to call the embryo artificial or unnatural. Such labels could only fit the artifacts used, such things as test tubes and lab (Petri) dishes.

The upshot of all this was that Dr. Petrucci later visited Soviet Russia and showed them his procedures. There he pushed his laboratory growth to double the number of cell divisions in his original experiment. Subsequently (in 1966), Dr. Pyotr Anakhin of the Academy of Medical Sciences in Moscow claimed that his team had kept 250 embryos going even longer—in one case for six months, to a weight of one and one-half pounds. But the Russian work, like Petrucci's original experiments, was never fully and acceptably reported, and remains in a "cloud of unknowing."

Dr. Rock had already done what Petrucci did, although for a shorter series of cell divisions. So had Dr. Landrum Shettles of the Columbia University College of Physicians and Surgeons in the 1950s. However, Shettles had never tried to see how long he could grow an embryo artificially *in vitro*. To show how real the moral issues are, when Dr. Shettles attended an International Fertility Conference in Italy in 1954, Pope Pius publicly condemned those who "take the Lord's work into their own hands."

In 1971, Shettles was the first investigator to actually implant an artificial or laboratory conceptus in a woman's womb, doing it at the implantable or "blastocyst" stage of sixty-five or more cell divisions (about five days' growth). That particular patient was to have a hysterectomy in another day or two anyway, because of cancer of the cervix. The egg transfer was done only to see if it would nidate, which it did; it was not done to bring it to birth. Shettles plans to embark on the "for keeps" procedure soon.

Across the Atlantic in England two medical researchers, Dr. Patrick Steptoe and Dr. Robert Edwards, have announced that they are ready to do an egg transfer, either a woman's own or one from a donor. This will not be done just as a pure experiment but as a therapeutic effort clinically. Needless to say, their work, like Shettles', is being closely followed in the scientific media, although reporters have poor luck getting them to talk about it. The English physicians are planning to insert the conceptus into the patient's uterus by a laparascope, a slender tube through the abdominal wall, but it is understood that Dr. Shettles intends to do his by the vaginal-cervix entry—as in artificial insemination of sperm. AI is already a current practice, and ET could easily become one too before this book is off the press. The Steptoe-Edwards team has more than fifty patients waiting, mostly married women.

When the problem of immunosuppression is solved it will be possible to replace by transplants all defective parts of the reproductive system—ovaries, testes, uteruses, tubes. Meantime, while the antibody mechanism stands in the way, there are still a number of options. If a woman has had her Fallopian tubes taken out or closed off irreversibly she could still have a baby by artificially taking an egg from her ovary and inseminating it with her husband's sperm or somebody else's *in vitro*, then implant it in her womb. If her tubes were blocked by disease the same procedure would fit her case. Even if not only the tubes were dysfunctioned but her ovaries as well, from sterility or an ovarian disease, she could still have her baby fathered by her husband by having a donated ovum fertilized with his sperm and then implanting it in her womb.

Another reason for an egg transfer (from a donor) might be the patient's serious genetic defects. Or if she is unable to interrupt her career outside the home in order to complete a pregnancy, as may become the case more often in these days of women's liberation, she could have her baby by surrogation; her egg and her husband's or lover's seed could be combined *in vitro* and implanted in another woman's uterus until brought to birth.

The same procedure would fit the case of a woman dying of carcinoma or leukemia who may want to leave *her* child behind her fathered by her husband or lover. Either hostess or artificial gestation could be resorted to. If she was already pregnant before her fate was discovered she could have her embryo transferred to a surrogate or to a glass womb, preserving the fetus even though she herself had to die. It is already being done with animals.†

† A bundle of ethical and legal questions are raised. For example, could the hostess claim to be the true mother? It also invites coarse humor about "wombs for rent" and the like, especially from those whose motive for their jokes is antagonism to the mode itself. These were ever the growing pains and problems of humanistic achievement.

The banking of human sperm (and ova) some day soon is an important part of the new reproductive technologies. It got its start in 1953 at the University of Arkansas when three successful pregnancies were reported from frozen sperm. Five years later there was another series of twenty more quite normal children. Since then many babies (estimates vary but they are in the hundreds) have been conceived with frozen sperm. Usually ejaculates are diluted in a protective fluid, sealed and stored in thirty to forty plastic straws, clustered in a cigar-shaped aluminum container in liquid nitrogen at −321 degrees Fahrenheit.‡ One clinic charges $25 a year storage per specimen, and a sperm bank's charge is likewise figured to be around $25 a year. Banking was first done only in medical centers, for much shorter periods, for relatively immediate clinical use.

But nowadays long-term storage by such commercial banks as the Idant Corporation and Genetic Laboratories is getting started, based on success with animals. Healthy calves have been produced with sperm stored as long as eighteen years. Women have been impregnated with human sperm frozen for as long as two and a half years. Dr. Edward Tyler of UCLA reported to the American Medical Association in June 1971 that of a series of sixty-five children born this way only one child had an abnormality (a finger missing), which is altogether in line with general morbidity rates.

There are reservations, however, in some quarters until things are worked out more fully. The American Public Health Association has warned against oversimple expectations and possible abuses by commercial

‡ Freeze *drying* is being investigated too. A stimulus came recently from Russian geochemists who reported finding microorganisms 250 million years old (Paleozoic) in potassium rock in the Urals; they came to life or were reactivated in distilled water.

banks, and most fertility clinics are still using only fresh semen—from husbands and donors. The APHA has expressed a doubt whether human sperm will retain its potency longer than sixteen months in storage, and even if this is not accurate there is at least some loss of motility of stored sperm. In any case, for the present at least there are time limits on storing sperm, as there will be on ova when that process is worked out.

The major reason for freeze storing sperm thus far has been to help couples who wish to postpone pregnancies for two or three years. If the man is sterilized they can be sure to avoid unintended conceptions, and when they are ready the woman can have his store inseminated artificially. With others it is a kind of fertility insurance against the risks of losing one's children through death or divorce. A man in Minnesota was so concerned about his posterity (a fear that his son might be infertile) that he stored his own sperm, hoping that if his worst fears came true his daughter-in-law would accept an artificial insemination with it.

Semen or sperm banking has been proposed as a guard against radiation damage from nuclear attack or accident, or because a person's vocation is mortally dangerous. Some crewmen on atomic submarines are said to have done this, and some scientists engaged in nuclear physics and fuel research. At last women will be able to have a child by a spouse or lover long after his death, or when great distances separate them; it will be true for men too when ova are successfully frozen. It is even recommended that people of recognized beauty or brains, or some other notable strength, should contribute their seed to central banks for those who might want their genetic value.

When people select the germ cells of famous donors,

maybe a great scientist or artist or theater beauty, it is important to explain to them that it is not the famous one's seed that is important but the famous one's *parents'* seeds. An interesting case of male chauvinism appeared when a sperm bank official said it is not the famous *man's* sperm that counts but his *father's*. The fact is, of course, that an Einstein or an Elizabeth Barrett Browning are the product of a mother as well as a father, and equally importantly of environment and the individual's personal history. There is too much overly simple talk about direct inheritance from the donors in artificial inseminations and egg transfers.

The outlook is not only for banking unfertilized ova too, but of storing *fertilized* eggs—zygotes up to the blastocyst or uterine stage of development. Basic success has been reached experimentally at the Oak Ridge National Laboratory in Tennessee, where they have superovulated and fertilized mouse embryos, freezing them in long-term storage and then implanting them for womb nurture. Not only will couples be able someday to store their own conceptuses but conceptus donors can contribute (paid or unpaid) to couples in whom there is a mutual sterility or uncorrectable genetic hazard.

As contraception reduces the number of unwanted children for adoption childless people will resort more and more to donated sperm, ova, and zygotes. Banking ova will eliminate the need of repeated surgical extractions of eggs for egg transfers, from wife or donor. As the battle for immunity suppression drives ahead it will be easier to transplant ovaries and donated tubes, not only eggs. Testicles could be transplanted too, obviating the need to go to sperm banks or to have a direct (fresh) artificial insemination from a donor.

What They Call Cloning

Thus far we have been looking at donor-recipient sharing of sperm and eggs and conceptuses, but there is a fourth kind close at hand—body cell donors. This is essentially what cloning is. A fertilized ovum or zygote is extracted from the oviduct and the fertilizing done *in vitro*. Next, its nucleus is removed (enucleated) and a body or "somatic" cell is donated—sliced off or excised from a nonsexual part of a man or woman's body (it makes no difference which part)—and inserted in the original nucleus' place. Then the renucleated ovum is finally implanted in the uterus of its ovulator or a surrogate's, or (prospectively) in an artificial womb.

This procedure is called asexual or nonsexual because the baby produced from it is not the result of a combination of male and female germ cells. The body cell may itself be the result of sexual reproduction but now it is alone the starting point of a new individual; it does not combine with any other person's sex cell. People born of cloning may in turn donate *their* body cells in another round of cloning, or return to the sexual mode of fertilization, or both.

The child produced in this way has all of his genetic inheritance solely from the body cell—that is, he will have only the genotype of the person whose body cell was used, invariably including the same sex. The new individual has one parent only, not two, and—what is more—is that parent's identical twin. Such cloned individuals, however, would be entirely fertile if their father or mother was, and able in their own turn to reproduce either sexually or asexually.

In a recent religious argument one antagonist said

he would believe in ordaining women for the ministry only when it became possible for a man to produce a child. To him such a thing seemed impossible, but it is not. The old saying was that all life is *ex ova*, from eggs, but this is no longer true. Children could be produced with a father and no mother, or a mother and no father. The DNA in every one of our body cells is the master tape of an entire genetic inheritance—it does not need other tapes to be reproduced.

In the language of reproductive science this procedure or method is called vegetative replication. Its precedent or model occurs in animal and plant husbandry, as well as in simple bacterial organisms. For example, it is done with carrots and tobacco, and with fruit flies, salamanders, frogs, and mice. There are no theoretical obstacles to human cloning and the technical problems may be rapidly surmounted. It is common to hear it predicted for humans by 1980—regardless of whether such prophets like it or frown on it.

Even cloning from the dead is possible. If a man or woman died before they had reproduced or, as the lawyers like to say, without issue, a cell cutting could be taken from their body (if it is done soon enough, before "cell death" takes place some hours after the brain and heart cease working) and replicated in any of the various modes or methods already described. If both husband and wife die, maybe in an auto or airplane wreck, it could be done—they could each have a child, thus preserving posterity and inheritance for both of them. If one or the other or both had a genetic disease or handicap that ethically ruled out sexual reproduction they could clone from the "clean" one or from a donor. A sterile woman could get an egg from another woman, have it renucleated with one of her own body cells, then have it implanted in her own uterus and "carry" it to term. Or if her husband was sterile she could receive an egg, her own or another's, renucleated with *his* body cell so that he might have a son of his own genetically. Its constructive uses are manifold.

The word "clone" comes from a Greek word meaning a sprout or slip or cutting. When a slip from a tree is planted in the ground it grows asexually, without fertilization, into the same thing—at least genetically, for environment makes many physical differences. It is the same with slips or clones of living tissue when they are planted in *their* appropriate ground—human tissue, the container egg. The word is used also as a verb, "to clone," even though Webster's thus far has given it only the nominative form.**

Wild Talk

It is foolish to talk, as some have, as if we could make "Xerox copies" or "carbon copies" of people simply by cloning them, or by genetic designing with the insertion, deletion, and transduction of genes and chromosomes. Somebody years ago in one of the liberal weeklies pointed out that a man might have his son's height "tailored" genetically to be a tall basketball player and then find that the boy wanted to play chess. Talk about cloning dozens of Einsteins or Hitlers and of how it would stunt the personal growth of a child to know he was an exact copy of somebody else is bogeyman talk. Toffler in *Future Shock* was

** Actually *a clone* is a company or group and it is not strictly accurate to use the word for individual cases of somatic replication. Webster's Second defines it as "The aggregate of individual organisms descended by asexual reproduction from a single sexually produced individual."

being properly careful when he said "man will be able to make *biological* carbon copies of himself."[12] Even identical twins can be as unlike as pull and push.

Without claiming that anybody is exactly unique we can see how variable the patterns of life and conditioning are, even within the same genetic structure and the same culture and social setting. Unique genotypes and unique environments interact to produce unique individuals in unique ways. Even a cloned (nonunique) genotype forms a unique individual as it interacts with its own "history."

This personal variety within genetic unity is due not only to minute or huge differences in the individual's growth and experience but also to the fact that genetically our traits or tendencies are set by a *bundle* of genes. This fact is what is called the polygenic nature of traits such as intelligence, temperament, and physique. They are not simple one-gene effects. Only a few traits in us are monogenic. Most of the things that give us identity as individuals are the results of polygenic combinations.

The point can be made by looking at intelligence. To determine a child's intelligence quotient (I.Q.) genetically would mean first identifying and then manipulating thousands of genes in a very complicated submicroscopic system. The very thought is mind boggling. It is certainly beyond any presently imaginable capability. Some geneticists, even including the eminent H. J. Muller, have talked rather wildly about selecting genotypes to improve not only intelligence but even character. Think also of the wide range of differences people acquire through their individual experience. We are familiar with the palpable differences between identical twins, even in controlled and identical situations.

The theory is advanced that certain racial groups

have a lower intelligence level than others (a very questionable thesis) and that this is due to genetic differences (much more questionable). Even if the theory were correct it could mean only a *statistical* difference and would say nothing whatsoever about the I.Q.'s of individuals in any racial group.[13] Once the "fast draw" critics of cloning appreciate the polygenic and "polyenvironmental" nature of most personality profiles, to say nothing of the polymorphic nature of even single gene traits, they will have to drop all their nonsense about Xerox and carbon copies.

There are, of course, other ways to control intelligence besides the control of health care, diet, stimulus, motivation, and learning. The brain's *size* might be increased, for example, thus raising the I.Q. Chemical treatment may be found to do it. At present the human brain reaches nine billion cells in the fetal cerebral cortex with thirty-three divisions, but with a thirty-fourth division the brain power would be tremendous.†† But since this would make the head too big at birth for the birth canal (it is already too big for comfortable delivery), the only answer would be the glass womb. All that limits I.Q. now, as far as its neurologic apparatus is concerned, is the size of the pelvis.

Quality control in birth technology will have to aim at selecting for intelligence and, where possible, lifting it. What any of us learns is not inherited but our *capacity* to learn is. In the past era of fast and indiscriminate population growth there has been a nega-

†† Human beings start with a single fertilized cell containing only one double set of genes, but it only takes forty-six successive divisions to reach thirty-five trillion cells. Such is the magnitude of geometric or exponential growth. One divides into two, two into four, four into eight, eight into sixteen, sixteen into thirty-two, thirty-two into sixty-four—and this makes only a mere six divisions.

tive correlation between mental ability and fertility. After all, if the new birth technology simply saves any and all babies—even those of very defective quality which would formerly have died *in utero* or after birth —it is a questionable achievement. It would be a disastrous instance of the dysgenic paradox of medicine, by which the gain in quantity brings with it a loss of quality.

There are more than three and a half billion people in the world. It took from the beginning of human history to 1830 for the world population to reach its first billion. The second billion was added in a single century. The third has taken only thirty years. The fourth billion will be reached by 1975—in only fifteen years' time. Death control, especially mass sanitation and disease prevention, has not been balanced by equally effective birth control.

Women between the ages of fifteen and fifty can have as many as twenty children. To have fewer obviously calls for some kind of conception prevention and birth prevention. A further potential hazard in the way of population and quality control is indicated by studies showing that menarche (the onset of menstruation and fertility) has dropped in Western countries from age seventeen about one hundred years ago to age thirteen today. And menopause has been postponed from age forty-five to fifty.

Population and Social Quality

Contraception and selective fetal control, backed by genetics; this "troika" is the only possible policy in a ZPG era—a time when "zero population growth" is a necessity if we are ever to halt the pollution and murder of our environment, to say nothing of the density which destroys our peace and quiet.

The cover of the U.S. family planning stamp for its first day (March 18, 1972) showed a portrait of Margaret Sanger saying, "No woman can call herself free . . . until she can choose whether or not to be a mother." It was over fifty years ago that she published her first controversial article, in 1912, and opened the first birth control clinic in 1916. Women have indeed "come a long way," and so has reproductive medicine.

In the period 1966–70, according to the findings of a national fertility survey by the Population Council in Princeton, there were 2,650,000 unplanned babies born. Unplanned babies are not necessarily unwanted; some became wanted, happily for them, but the cost socially and psychologically is very high. Over 40 per cent of our human reproduction was unplanned. "Population and the American Future," the report of the presidential commission chaired by John D. Rockefeller, Jr., recommended three major policies: (1) free access to birth control for minors as well as adults; (2) free voluntary sterilization; and (3) freedom of abortion in the first two trimesters if personally requested and medically administered.

These proposals reflect a most important change of ethical opinion in America. In 1968, only 15 per cent favored freedom of abortion in the Gallup polls but by 1972 it had climbed to 64 per cent over-all, including a majority (56 per cent) of Catholics. Even among people with less than a high school education there were 47 per cent in favor, 45 per cent opposed. As to contraconceptive guidance for minors there was an over-all vote of 73 per cent in favor, which reached 87 per cent among college people.[14] This was backed by a U. S. Supreme Court decision in 1972 declaring unconstitutional a Massachusetts law which had denied contraception to unmarried persons.

Some minority groups protested the Rockefeller commission's report, moved by religious beliefs or requirements. The Catholic bishops called it as a whole an "ideological valley of death." The Missouri Synod Lutherans remained silent about the abortion part but joined in the Catholic bishops' condemnation of the report. A few politicians got on the religious bandwagon for vote-getting reasons. Nevertheless, the report has the future written all over it, in spite of the ideological fury it faced at first.

III

SOME DOUBTS

We claimed earlier that ignorance of the essential facts about birth biology makes us part of the problem itself, rather than of its solution. By the same token, to be ignorant of the doubts and objections felt by people in the "resistance forces" would also undermine our ability to cope with the problem.

We often tell our children that in defending any opinion or policy they ought to know what the objections are—and, what is more, they should be able to state those objections to the objector's satisfaction. It behooves us, then, to take a good close look at the reservations, criticisms, reactions, and complaints commonly raised against the new reproductive medicine. Later we can take a good *hard* look at their merits.

In prescientific times the whole subject of trying to "breed supermen" or "man making man" by other than the natural sexual process was a favorite one for myth makers. Their myths reveal how ambivalent and conflicted people are about it.[1] Doctor Faustus tried it by the philosophers' stone; in Goethe's version he did it with Homunculus in the phial. The Icelandic sagas used androids to express the half-and-half feeling of being both man and animal. Prometheus tried to make men like gods and came a cropper. The Talmud treated the golem or half men with obviously ambivalent and even contradictory judgment. The Cabalists did too.

In more modern myths, Mary Shelley's Frankenstein ended in tragic failure and so did Karel Čapek's
robots in *R.U.R.* The key to all such mythology is,
be it noted, man's wondering not only about the
"secret of life" but whether it is *morally* proper for
him to want to know it. Paracelsus, the alchemist, got
both good and bad marks in the traditional literature;
some sent him to hell for his arrogance, others allowed
him final salvation and credit.

Fear of Consequences

The general public is more apt to have doubts than
those who are closer to the biological frontier. Inquiries into the values and moral attitudes of physicians and scientists show that they sometimes have
technical doubts about the discoverability or workability of some of the new biology's goals, but that they
find relatively little in the way of basic moral objections. Their usual test for whether anything like
egg transfers or ectogenesis is desirable or not is how
much it promises to cure illness or promote health
and human well-being.[2]

Trying to do both of these things, to cure patients
and promote well-being, we can run into complications. Some things are therapeutic in particular cases
but harmful generally. Other things are therapeutic
but nevertheless carry undesirable side effects or long-
term results which might outweigh the good they do.
Opiates are an example of the first kind of complica-
tion. The dysgenic effect of saving newborns with
pyloric stenosis—if they are allowed to survive and
spread it by sexual reproduction—could be an example
of the second kind.

Few people with medical and humane purposes,

however, would adopt the wedge argument. They are not willing to throw away good things because of the possibility (as distinguished from the certainty) of undesired entailments. Instead, their inclination would be to limit the opiates to medical uses, and to correct pyloric stenosis but prevent its carriers from reproducing—and to prevent it by either voluntary or, if necessary, compulsory controls. Rather than the wedge objection, a kind of all-or-nothing distortion of the virtue of prudence, men of science and medicine follow the classical ethical guideline of "the proportionate good."

Some objections are posed in an *a priori* and doctrinaire way, some more pragmatically. Some are whole-hog objections, some are measured and weighed up relatively in a pro-and-con fashion. Some are highly subjective; some quite objective.

Dr. Robert Gorney, psychiatrist at the UCLA Medical School, is one of the more pragmatic and relativistic kind of question askers, a critical thinker in the true sense of the word.[3] He indicates some of the mental and emotional hurdles and growing pains foreseeable in the new birth technologies. But he does not cry, "Halt!" He wants us to consider the "possible dismal results" of the new reproductive medicine and to carefully examine the trade-off problems of genetic control, weighing the desirable against the undesirable. This is all in a sturdy effort to be clinical, rather than universalizing prohibitions. He judges these things in terms of their consequences, not by an *a priori* rejection based on nontherapeutic grounds.

At one extreme we find a writer who feels that such treatments as artificial insemination, egg transfers, and nuclear transplants are "an assault on . . . marriage and the human family," flatly rejecting any idea that we should try to "produce optimum babies" (the best possible). Furthermore, he argues that those who justify the artificial methods introduced by biomedical technology are "family wreckers" and that such techniques are depersonalizing and dehumanizing. Basically he argues that the arts of medical "manufacture" (artificial reproduction) bypass the "mystery of nature" and that the only legitimate mode of parenting is not only sexual but coital.[4]

On the other hand there are some question askers who only raise objections to particular procedures, without wholly condemning all of the new modes in a lump. In between, some are ready to approve of the therapeutic uses of the new biology but oppose anything like genetic engineering or designing. They can find a moral defense for remedial treatments but not for constructive manipulations of the elemental genetic "stuff" of a human being. We will look at some of the questions raised along this spectrum of doubt, from whole-hog condemnations to skeptical specifics.

A doubt of the more over-all kind was registered dramatically in 1970 when a twenty-six-year-old Harvard bacteriologist, James Shapiro, quit science and the whole genetics effort cold. He and two colleagues had just succeeded in isolating a pure gene for the first time. He explained that such work might be put to evil uses by governments and big corporations, that the "system" does not allow "the people" to have any say in what scientists are doing, and that things like stopping the Vietnam War and pollution are more important.

Respect For Life

A common doubt has to do with respect for human life. If we exercise a radical control over the sources of life will it not result in a kind of arrogant and contemptuous attitude? This is really a part of the wedge argument. Does it not cheapen life, the objection goes, to tailor it genetically, to start and stop it at will? Do we not degrade human life if we conceive it in laboratories or cultivate it in glass containers rather than in the human body? Is it not disrespectful of life to "manufacture" people by laboratory fertilization, for example, or by intervening in the gene structure and heredity of people? Will it not end, the objectors wonder with foreboding, in a world where sex is abolished and reproduction is carried on by cloning?

It is hard to take hold of a doubt like this one because it is so unobjective, so untied to any specific course of reasoning. The vitalist idea that life as such is sacrosanct, the highest good and somehow both sacred and untouchable, is obviously not tenable in actual practice. If we held to it consistently there would be no ethical basis for heroism or martyrdom or even of killing in self-defense. Like all such absolutes and universals it is constantly contradicted by those who preach it, even though some of them preach it with utter sincerity. For example, vitalists are very apt at the same time to defend capital punishment and military killing, along with "justifiable homicide" in a myriad of situations.

If their first concern was for *persons*, living people with minds and personalities, their moral inconsistencies would perhaps not be so obvious, but to hold as they do that *life* as such, and at any stage of development and quality, is untouchable runs into too many reasonable exceptions to stand up as a moral rule. An ideal, yes; a rule, no.

As an ideal, respect for life would be challenged by very few, if by anybody. Even Schopenhauer with all his pessimism urged only quietism, not suicide. But ideals are subject to all sorts of exceptions and qualifications on a trade-off or tit-for-tat basis. The problem arises when we are confronted with a choice between having a defective baby or an abortion; between remaining ignorant of how to take care of fetuses or gaining the required knowledge by starting and stopping ("killing") conceptuses; between choosing childlessness or resorting to artificial reproduction; between accepting the exhaustion of the environment or having population control; between having an increasingly polluted gene pool and exerting genetic control; between voluntary or compulsory pregnancy. And so on.

There is nothing helpful in such heavy-handed humor as Jacob Bronowski's at a 1963 conference about the genetic control of inherited defects. Referring to Swift's satirical *Modest Proposal* he said, "Indeed, we might achieve the same effect in a simpler way—by eating the children of the unfit, as Jonathan Swift suggested that the Irish poor should eat their own children."[5]

For example, respect for life and the love of children are usually tied together. But if there is any moral obligation to have children it must be relative to population and natural resources. Respect for environment and for life as a whole has claims just as real as the desire for more children. It is absurd to ignore the radical difference between the problems of population in the agricultural-rural society of the past and the industrial-urban society of today. In the present era with its lowered mortality rate and density of dwelling we cannot and *should* not keep to the old biblical piety "Be fruitful and multiply," without some careful calculation and control.

As Dr. Paul Pruyser of the Menninger Clinic says,

"To take this text out of context and turn it into an everlasting moral injunction is a pernicious form of fundamentalism" because it cuts across the "new ethic of reproduction" we need in order to survive.[6] The Bible makes no mention of any "right" to choose family size or to not reproduce at all. Being "fruitful" was not a personal election; whether a woman was cursed with being barren or blessed with fertility was a matter of divine fiat, not of human control and responsibility. That is certainly no basis for a sane ethics.

We once had to multiply in order to survive; now we cannot survive if we do. People are beginning to feel the force of a remark by Dr. Littlefield: "The world no longer needs all the individuals we are capable of bringing into it—especially those who are unable to compete and are an unhappy burden to others. If the size of our families must be limited, surely we are entitled to children who are healthy rather than defective."[7]

Doubts based on "respect for life" remind us of the constant tension between a sanctity-of-life ethics and a quality-of-life ethics—two moral or value positions which are not only different but sometimes actually opposed to each other. This issue will surface time after time in what follows.

The respect-for-life objection is often tied psychologically to the feeling that mastery of life will kill its mystery and that the mystery of life is essential to respect for it. This attitude in turn reinforces the "stop meddling" attitude which favors blissful ignorance. If it were to dominate it would stifle or at least hobble not only biology but the chemistry on which biology is built.

People used to talk about the fact of life itself being a mystery. Back in the 1930s Harold Urey at the University of Chicago figured that ultraviolet radiation of the gases which make up the earth's atmosphere was what started life. In 1953 his student Stanley Miller set up a test experiment using simple gases such as ammonia, methane, hydrogen, and water vapor. It worked. Miller's test resulted in the "creation" of amino acids and nucleic acid bases—the building blocks of life. It is hard to believe, however, that this end to a mystery would of itself kill respect and awe of life. For many people of imagination and intellectual vigor it actually enhanced their appreciation. Respect that depends on ignorance is doomed.

The Proper Way to Propagate

There is a strong sentiment that it is somehow unnatural and "bad" to go outside of the coitus-gestation mode of reproduction. We might call this the proper-way-to-propagate thesis. More likely than not it arises from a strong sense of human romance and of the dynamic force of interpersonal relations. It may also come from a deep experience of the mutual commitment of a husband and wife in their love making and baby making, the historic and familiar nexus of the family.

After all, the phrase "in a family way" means far more than just being pregnant. It means a whole bundle of human ties and creative satisfactions. Will the new modes of reproduction undermine romantic and family love, even though they are hardly likely ever to be anything more than second choice to the natural mode? Could they not actually strengthen marriage in some situations? One objector asks if we want to eliminate "biological kinship"—although it should be obvious that it would be impossible to do so as long as we reproduce, whether we do it naturally or artificially.[8] What he really is asking is whether we are willing to eliminate sexual intercourse, and the answer should be obvious: "No. But we might be willing to reproduce another way in some situations."

Some psychologists and sociologists (and even some religiously oriented observers) believe it is a mistake ethically and humanly to equate being faithful in marriage with making it a sexual monopoly. Few of us any more look upon a husband or wife as property. Insemination or enovulation from a third-party donor is not an "invasion of monogamous marriage rights" if a couple agree in choosing it. If they understand their relationship morally and personally, rather than physically and sexually, the problem disappears. In the same vein, basing integrity and fidelity on personal relationship, we would regard an adopted child or one conceived by artificial insemination as being fully and truly one's child, whereas a battered or neglected child would *not* be its genetic parents' child even though they brought it into the world by coitus gestation.

The last sentence in one attack is "Have we enough sense to turn back?"—to which it might be answered, "No, not if we lack the sense to go ahead." People who feel as the objector does are apt to want a moratorium on reproductive science and medical research, or even to try to police or suppress them. There is a thin line somewhere at which the effort to politically control biological control will become the very dictatorship which the advocates of suppression are afraid of.

As Plato remarked (*Republic* I. 333), the same doctor who can keep us from disease would also be clever at producing it by stealth. The issue is whether human beings are to be trusted to use reproductive technology humanely. The critic we have just been reporting declares straightforwardly that noncoital reproduction is both dehumanizing and depersonalizing.

This charge is of the *a priori* kind; it simply asserts that artificial modes are *as such* immoral. But he also tries to reinforce his condemnation by claiming that artificial modes are subject to abuse, and this is argument of a different kind; it appeals to consequences which allegedly will or might follow from the practice.

Of the two kinds of moral argument, pragmatic reasoning based on consequences is more rational and discussable. Bland *a priori* assertions of opinion we cannot either verify or falsify. How can we possibly check out the dire predictions of abuse and misuse on which the don't-trust-human-beings objection is based? On the record human beings have used their knowledge for *both* good and evil, and it is sensible to suppose that this "double effect" will happen also with the new reproductive medicine.

The "parade of horrors" strategy, however, is an ax that cuts two ways. After all, it was the "good old natural way" that the Third Reich officials turned to in their racist program, when they established the Ordenburgen where Aryan youth were sent to make babies—babies that met the phenotypic selection standards of the Nazi blood-and-soil mystique. Furthermore, the Nazis' pseudoscientific experiments with genetics and the cruelties perpetrated by some of their doctors were neither genetic nor eugenic anyway; they were aimed at ethnic politics and genocide.[9] The remedy lies in a more humane politics, not in the paralysis of biology and medicine.

Tyranny will always use whatever means lie at hand —it certainly has never waited for artificial insemination and enovulation, nor for ectogenesis and cloning. New modes are subject to tyrannous use just as the old ones are. Most things are vulnerable to misuse, just as marriage itself is; in the language of the traditional religious ceremony, marriage ought not to be "entered into unadvisedly or lightly." In any case, however, the fear of tyranny is a big element among the Doubting Thomases and we must try to appreciate it.

Another version of the fear of risk is the claim that misuse of artificial modes will be *unintentional* but none the less objectionable. This appeal to ignorance of the future as a reason for remaining ignorant in the present is an age-old weapon in the armory of reactionaries. They say, for example, that we cannot be sure that eradicating genetic diseases will be a good thing; if we succeed it might have unforeseeable and far worse end results. This is hypothetically possible, to be sure, but only in the same way that it is dangerous to be alive. The danger *if we do not eradicate genetic diseases* is far more real and evident.

Our champion of CG-only follows up his attack by saying that the real danger comes not from the evildoers but the do-gooders. He is more afraid of "the well-wishers of mankind, for folly is much harder to detect than wickedness"—he concludes that the dangerous people are the ones who want to prevent the birth of defective babies and who talk about the quality of life.[10] There, in a few cruel words, the issue stands stark naked.

When a warning voice comes out of clinical caution, as compared to the coital-only champion's whole-hog back-to-nature reaction, we have solid cause to listen. Dr. R. D. Hotchkiss was well within the range of responsible thinking when he reminded us that in our concern for our gene pool we need to beware of "atomic fallout, overzealous X-raying, dilution by the prolific insane, and qualitative mishandling by the insanely optimistic."[11]

Another general doubt appears in the claim that human traits and qualities are far too polygenic to be controlled by genetic means. This is a you-cannot-do-the-good-you-want argument. It is certainly true that much more needs to be known and it may be true that not very much beyond control of single gene traits will ever be possible. The answer is not in yet, but not *wanting* it answered at all is merely self-crippling.

Almost diametrically opposed to this in logic is the objection that genetics will give *complete* control—turning people into robots or prefabricated automatons who will act out their designers' plans to the letter. This is a you-cannot-avoid-the-evil-you-do-not-want argument. Another form of this objection is based on our need for genetic variety, which is provided by sexual combination. Even the single cell paramecia have to "merge" with one another after a series of asexual reproductions, before they can resume their solo system. The fear is that selective genetic control might end us up in a fixed and invariable gene pool, producing only a few interchangeable types. This notion is probably inspired by Aldous Huxley's clever picture of fixed human types: alpha personalities, betas, gammas, deltas, and epsilons.

Some doubters doubt that genetic engineering will work while others have no doubt that it will work but they still doubt that it can serve humane purposes. The objection based on you *can* do it but shouldn't is worth a little closer look. Especially in certain religious circles it has been argued at great length (1) that individuality is of very great moral value, (2) that genetic controls—especially cloning—will prefabricate people right down to the minute details into preprogrammed creatures, just carbon or Xerox copies, and (3) that to practice designed or purposive reproduction wipes out individuality which, to be authentic, must be the result of sexual chance. In this kind of reasoning reproductive control is therefore morally wrong. In its simplest form it is a syllogism: Individuality is essential to humanity, genetic control destroys individuality, *ergo* genetic control is inhumane. Now nobody wants to be a rubber stamp; objection along this line may appear to carry some weight in the eyes of the unwary who accept its presupposition that engineering *personalities* can be done genetically. The presupposition is false.

We have already noted this. As the Canadian biologist N. J. Berrill says with an amused snort between the lines, "Artists cannot be counted on to breed artists, nor do astronomers breed astronomers. Nor can the inheritance of general intelligence be predicted. Unusually intelligent parents can produce human vegetables as readily as do other couples, while individuals of exceptional merit tend to crop up everywhere in ordinary run-of-the-mill families."[12]

To think in terms of genetic "copies" is what José Delgado calls "the error of potentiality."[13] Genetic replication does not equate with personality replication. The most that can be said is that similar or the same genotypes would *tend statistically* to result in a similar physical appearance and similar glandular or endocrine dispositions. That is, in a large enough spread of a given genetic "program" there would probably be a discernible incidence of traits of the sort that are made possible by the physical or physiological system set by the genes.

Nothing more than this can be said.* Dr. Berrill's humorous come-off-it statement, by the way, applies to clones as well as to mate-selected children. An in-

---

* "Preformation" was an old theory that everything about the individual was already present in the human seed. Spermists said that the little man or homunculus was in the sperm, ovists said he was in the egg. The opposite and equally mistaken doctrine of the "epigenetic" camp held that everything is due to the environment and experience—that the newborn is a *tabula rasa*. Neither position is tenable.

dividual cloned from Hitler could be a saintly school-teacher; one from Einstein could be a golf instructor or a bank robber. There is nothing in the bogeyman fear that power-mad tyrants could clone themselves as an elite and rule the world—on the model of Hitler and his *Übermenschen.*

Do No Harm

Still others have a fear of doing harm to people by these new birth technologies, especially while they are in their experimental or earlier stages. An old saying in medical ethics is *sed nil nocere* or *primum, non nocere.* These are the Latin words of a couple of versions of the Hippocratic oath (there are many other versions). It means that doctors cannot always help their patients but at least they ought not to do them any harm.

Some moralists include embryos among the "people" who might be hurt. They claim that we endanger actual human beings when we risk injuring an embryo during an *in vitro* fertilization or a subsequent implantation. They therefore oppose work like Shettles' and the English team Edwards and Steptoe's. Obstetricians, however, point out that some of the accidents feared can already be detected and such embryos aborted, that more will be discoverable as they progress, and that in any case there are no more congenital mishaps (if as many) in these artificial modes than in natural fertilizations and pregnancies. The English obstetrician R. F. R. Gardner, a professed Christian, calls it a "trivialization" to claim that spontaneously aborted conceptuses and *in vitro* conceptuses are human beings or persons or souls.[14]

Wise and humane as the principle of *non nocere* is, it cannot be a strict or universal rule. Surgery is an obvious exception to it. Medicine does its prescribing and treating with an unavoidable margin of uncertainty and risk and there are innumerable treatments which hurt as well as help, on a trade-off or "proportionate good" basis. This being so, medical ethics has always safeguarded the ideal of not doing harm with two further limiting principles. One is that any risks and injuries involved ought to be for the sick person's benefit, nobody else's; the other (its reverse) is that innocent third parties, people other than the patient, ought not to be victimized for the patient's sake.

It is pretty plain that an ethical code based on these general principles is going to run into practical difficulties. For example, it is almost impossible to carry out a scientifically sound clinical trial if you stick completely to the benefit principle; some of the patients involved will get a placebo or make-believe treatment, some will be given the outmoded treatment, still others will get the drug or treatment believed to be better. If such "double blind" tests are carried out widely enough to be valid there are bound to be some who suffer, either positively or negatively, for the sake of others. Even if "informed consent" is had from the patients participating, based on both knowledge of the risks and willingness to undergo them, there is still lack of benefit for some.

Several of Dr. Steptoe's patients are volunteers who know quite well that the attempt to do egg transfers (from the wife or from donors of the egg and/or sperm) may fail in their own case but they do it because it might help others. The voluntary principle obtains in all artificial inseminations and egg transfers and it will, presumably, be an ethical requirement also in artificial gestation and nuclear transplants. Even so, even when people undergo it willingly, some critics object to running any risk of their being hurt.

An even more extreme version of the do-no-harm doctrine insists that zygotes and embryos (not just patients) may be harmed and that it is therefore immoral to do either research or therapy involving any risk of harm—known or unknown and no matter how unintentional. A critic of this type says, "We cannot morally *get to know* how to perfect" artificial inseminations and implantations "unless the *possibility* of such damage can definitely be excluded" from *in vitro* procedures. This would bring it all to a dead stop. Extensive animal studies should be done first, of course, but at some point *they* must be confirmed by human trials—as in all medical research.

Explaining that if embryos are damaged they can be discarded does not get around this argument's roadblock. Its major premise is that an embryo is a patient, a person, and that to discard a defective embryo is murder. The other side of the coin is that we cannot eliminate the possibility of damaged or defective natural or *in vivo* fertilizations either. Natural processes often damage the conceptus, so that the logic of the objection is to challenge both kinds of reproduction —the natural as well as the artificial.

Some objectors are prepared to go a lot further than this. They object on the ground that the embryos involved cannot give and have therefore not given their consent. Consent, they contend, is ethically required from every subject in investigative medicine. Not just from existing persons or patients, be it noted, but even from nonexisting or only potential persons. *In vitro* fertilizations, whether for experimental or therapeutic purposes, are ruled out because an embryo is obviously incapable of giving either willing or informed consent to anything.[15]

The assumption here, the main bone of contention in the abortion debate, is that embryos are persons. One religious moralist has argued that since "the unmade child" or "possible future human being" obviously cannot consent "he" (it) is not a volunteer and "before his beginning he† is in no need of a physician to learn how not to harm him."[16]

A cohort puts it in slightly changed language. It is wrong, he asserts, ever to use children in medical experiments but this condemnation applies "with even greater force" to experiments on "a hypothetical child (whose conception is as yet only intellectual)." This language has a somewhat Through-the-Looking-Glass unreality about it, basically because these moralists have saddled themselves with the claim that prenatal life is as human as anybody's and are trying to argue consistently with it. The absurdity of their objection is appreciated simply by remembering that babies produced in the coital-gestational or natural way could not have given *their* consent either. Which leaves us where?

Consistently enough the do-no-harm objection is also raised against amniocentesis, fetological therapy, egg transfers, artificial gestation, cloning—against all "manipulation" of reproduction. There is to be sure a marginal risk of injury in all of these things, just as there is in every other kind of medical treatment. But this is not a very weighty line of objection to artificial methods of reproduction for the simple reason that a similar margin of risk is equally true of raw nature's way of making babies. Errors certainly occur in both sexual and asexual forms of reproduction when they take place in nature and without rational controls.

† Observe the androcentric use of male or masculine pronouns.

Risk and error are always given factors; they exist in the very finiteness of things. And the point about artificial control is precisely that *it tends to reduce risk and error*, and is intended to do so.

Many of these protests are hardly more than mood expressions, feelings tied for the most part to traditional customs and values. They are *a priori*, not pragmatic; they are not conclusions based on a balance of good and evil consequences. Yet they are none the less influential.

However, besides such generalized objections there are also a number of specific challenges of specific aspects of the new reproductive medicine. Suppose we look at some of the more interesting ones.

In spite of ominous population pressures many people are still naïvely pro-natalist; they assert that they have a *duty* to have children. This is much the same thing as their saying they have a "right" to have children. The duty is usually said to be imposed by God's will (often Genesis 1:18 is cited: Be fruitful and multiply), and the right in support of the obligation is said to be implied.

As a matter of fact there is nothing in the Bible or in the literature of the past about restricting reproduction to the coital-gestational mode. The possibility simply never occurred to the moralists of the past —that there is any alternative—just as overpopulation never figured in their ethics. It is arguable, in any case, that if "procreation" *is* a duty it can be fulfilled by artificial modes as well as by the natural one. But the main point surely is that we cannot profitably turn for guidance to traditional morality on reproduction for the simple reason that the tradition makers were in utter ignorance of the options and of the realistic judgments called for by the options.

Third Party Help with Conception

When we look at more specific objections to specific techniques we find some startling ones. Artificial or therapeutic insemination has come in for its full share.[17] None of the objections to it is new but some of them are pressed with rising heat. Catholic theology condemns artificial insemination (donor) on the ground that a donor's seed is an intrusion into the monopoly of monogamy.‡ Artificial insemination from a donor is immoral, it is argued, no matter how generous or humane the motive, no matter how impersonal and nongenital the means; marriage is morally an exclusive sexual relationship between husband and wife. Sperm and ova are as much a part of a person's sex as their genitalia. *Ergo*, artificial insemination from a donor is immoral and a child thus conceived is a bastard. The same logic applies to enovulations.

This objection raises important questions in a new context about the nature of relationship, about marital fidelity, and about neighbor love and human helpfulness. All Catholics do not "buy" the official syllogism. For example, the embryologist Robert Francoeur is unwilling to narrow the range of parental and marital fidelity to such a "physicalist" or genitalized definition.[18] To the contrary, he reasons that not only is noncoital sexual intercourse justifiable but that there is no good case any more for "the reduction of fidelity

‡ These theologians allow artificial insemination with the husband's seed as "assisted" insemination *post coitum*, i.e., using the male fluid only if it is ejaculated in married coitus, but they ban "total AI" even if it is the husband's seed that is used. In short, sexual intercourse by coitus is essential to licit reproduction and it must always be within marriage. A similar position is taken by Orthodox Jews.

to a very simplistic but nicely black-and-white prohibition of coitus with anyone other than one's spouse."

The writer cited earlier, who objects to artificial enovulations because the fertilized ova have not given their consent, likewise objects to donor insemination on the same ground that the establishment Catholics do—that it is not morally lawful because it is not coital and marital; that monogamous marriage and sexual intercourse are "the limits of specifiably legitimate conduct" in reproduction.[19] As a religious opinion he further claims that donor insemination "means a refusal of the image of God's creation in our own," and that "the same Lord . . . presides over procreation as well as . . . marital covenants."

Here we have a well-defined syndrome of attitudes and alleged divine sanctions. It condemns every one of the artificial modes except "assisted husband's insemination." All of them are proscribed, as such. The objection is not to their use in particular cases or situations, for extrinsic reasons such as inappropriateness in a particular patient's physical or psychological condition. No, the objection is that they are intrinsically and inherently wrong, as being what they are.

Their condemnation is *a priori*, not based upon a pragmatic consideration of the consequences.** The religionist we have been quoting says flatly, in another place, that "there must be a determination of the rightness or wrongness of the action and not only of the good to be obtained in medical care or from medical investigation."[20] It is not the good that medicine does, he is saying, which makes a treatment right; its morality must be determined apart from the human benefit in terms of what is believed and felt about it.

** One way to condemn new things is to use fiction to portray only a disastrous case while ignoring successful ones. This is done in novels about "test tube fathers" and the like.

As we have seen, this is the basic question in all moral decision making; do we act according to consequences or according to religious and folk beliefs?

A few years ago a law providing for the new medical practice of therapeutic insemination was passed in the Oklahoma legislature, and during the debate the usual syndrome of objections was set forth by the opposition. Donor insemination, they said, (1) treats humans like cattle, (2) is a form of adultery, and (3) anyway, it may be God's will that some people should be childless.

The first objection is attitudinal, a mood position. The second objection is specific enough, even though debatable. Since the common law tradition never imagined that parenting can be achieved by means other than coital conception it has nothing to say about questions of the legitimacy, status, and rights of inheritance for children born by donor insemination, egg transfer, or nuclear transplant.

The third objection is the most alien and inimical to medicine because medicine's business is to help and cure. The theological spookery shown in the idea of special providence and divine favoritism is about what we would expect from people who are not ashamed to argue that humane goals are *not* the main concern of medical morality.

What about the incest objection—the warning that insemination from anonymous donors or from sperm banks will mean that some conceptions will fall within some prohibited range of family relationships? This applies also to egg transfers from donors of ova and sperm. The taboo on incest is strong in some communities and ethnic groups, even though we know now that the taboo is a matter of cultural bias and not of a sound biology.

Degrees of consanguinity (blood relationship) are

old hat as an objection, but the objection might now be based on geneticity or a "too close" genetic relationship. Actually, inbreeding is not biologically harmful except in family stocks too poor genetically to tolerate any accentuation of their genotypes. The strength of superior inbreeding is seen in famous instances like Moses, Cleopatra, the Ptolemies, and the ancient Egyptian ruling class; and the ruling family of Siam, who gave up incestuous reproduction only a couple of generations ago.

Nonetheless the taboo is strong. Like Pauling's mention of tattoo marks for bad gene carriers, Dr. Gorney thinks that if artificial insemination was more widely practiced we might have to wear "coded dog tags" to indicate our parenty and to avoid mating with a half sister or half brother.[21] At present the policy is to keep the donor's identity unknown, which opens the way to innocent combinations of bad genes. There may be good reasons for changing that policy, psychological as well as biological. But the fear of incest as such is not a rational objection.

Ann Landers once ran a question in her column touching on the marriage and incest hang-ups. It went like this. A sterile husband asks his wife to have an artificially conceived baby from his own father's sperm. The father-in-law says that only this would bring him to make their child his heir. She agrees about an AID but not to that particular source, explaining that while she admired her father-in-law she would have "strange feelings" about it. The columnist's reply made no objections to the procedure as such, only to the donor; she thought that in this particular case it might be self-emasculation psychologically on the husband's part. Her advice to the wife was not to give birth to her own "brother-in-law." Here we have a specific case in which it could indeed be a serious mistake, but to so diagnose it does not immoralize artificial insemination itself.

A few women, in the advance guard of a new kind of parenting and child rearing now emerging in the revolt against marriage peonage have had children by donor insemination. Bachelor women will soon be able to outwit inovulency as well as singleness; they will have egg transfers. And any woman with a reason to avoid pregnancy can someday arrange artificial gestation.

Quite apart, however, from these artificial aids or alternatives to conventional childbearing, and quite apart from the charge that they are immoral, another objection is raised—namely, that it is wrong for un-married people to have and rear children. It is even argued that unmarried couples, cohabiting immorally or illegally, would have at least a better right to chil-dren than bachelor parents do. The same objection is made to bachelor fathers. It makes news every time a child placement agency arranges an adoption for a bachelor, and a public debate follows. Lesbians bear-ing children without having to engage in heterosexual intercourse is a prospect which outrages many people.

With some the objection is as we have seen, *a priori*; only coital-gestational reproduction within the mar-riage bond is right. With others the objection is prag-matic and consequential; for example, it is contended that children are best brought up by a man and a woman together, having both gender figures in the pic-ture. While it may be admitted that many children grow up well without a father or a mother and that divorces are often sought to free children from one or the other parent, these situations—the argument runs —ought not to be designed deliberately, only endured when they happen to be the best way out.

Warnings Galore

The danger-of-doing-harm objection to laboratory assisted reproduction, especially egg transfers, is sometimes reinforced with other warnings. Are we going to make poor women into a childbearer caste while rich women go skiing? Would substitutes in gestation not be just hot houses, human incubators? One writer has called it "child buying and selling." (An English embryologist has actually suggested $5,000 as a good fee, when an actress cannot take maternity leave from her play, or the like.) Suppose the surrogate mother who carries another's child to term refuses to give it up? This is a possibility, of course. The psychological problem is not insurmountable, however, and the legal question will fairly promptly be settled.

The law at present has no guidelines as between the claims of the conceiver and the gestator because it has always assumed coitus-gestation to be the only possible mode of reproduction. It is also said darkly that women who are willing to bear children for others may be disordered psychologically, and this, too, could be the case. It certainly can be and often is true of "normal" mothers. The normal is not the natural, nor vice versa.

Objection to natural or human incubators, which is what surrogates are, is equaled and sometimes exceeded by objection to artificial gestation. Little is said against it rationally but the feeling against it is often very strong. This happens in spite of our familiarity over a long time with incubators for premature deliveries in cases of uterine or fetal pathologies, whether the "preemies" come by spontaneous or induced delivery.

The prospect of having an open window on a growing fetus is welcomed by most of those in responsible roles—embryologists, placentologists, fetologists. Their chance to monitor fetal life in the light, out of the darkness and obscurity of the womb, will add enormously to our knowledge and help us reduce the hazards that face obstetricians and their patients. We realize that the womb is a dark and dangerous place, a hazardous environment. We should want our potential children to be where they can be watched and protected as much as possible.

The objection is that this is "unnatural." And if physicians or scientists using the glass womb to monitor or manipulate fetal tissue find reasons to end it before it reaches term, for whatever reason, whether experimental or therapeutic, they bump up against the "murder" charge. With the morphon (shape) of the fetus so plainly in view the "homunculus reaction" is also apt to be stronger than ever; we see this in some young nursing and medical students when they are suddenly shown a bottled fetus in an anatomy laboratory or a pathology department.

Nuclear transplants or what is called "renucleation" or cloning runs into a lot of objections. It is perhaps more widely attacked than the assisted modes of sexual reproduction we have been considering. One nonbiologist calls it a "freak" phenomenon. To have a child solely in one person's genetic "image" is called a genetic narcissism, as surely it could be in some cases. We have already looked at the carbon-copy objection to it; groundless as it is it continues to be perpetrated. A similar scare cry is that cloned individuals are dead ends biologically. The fact is, of course, that cloned people can reproduce sexually as well as by another cloning, and if it is done sexually their partners too can be either cloned or of sexual origin. Cloning is a particular mode of reproduction for particular cases; it can alternate with sexual reproduction as need suggests, in one generation or another.

It has been argued that the clones or clonant will be more resentful than an identical twin is—because the twin is at least born naturally of a double fertilization. This greater resentment of the cloned person, the argument runs, will stem from the knowledge that unlike twinning their being cloned is deliberate and designed. One or two critics have tried to buttress this consequential objection with the *a priori* assertion that everybody has a right to a "unique genotype." Deducing from that doctrinaire assumption, the argument is that a twin loses his right through no one's fault but a clonant has been deliberately deprived of it. The point is then, that twinning is tragic but cloning is malicious.

The counter consideration here, obviously, is that all identical twins do not feel this way about it, and there is no reason to assume that all clonants will feel that way either. It is a factor to be weighed up with other factors, that is all. It has even been declared in a bizarre kind of psychology that the cloned individual will have no "free will," no independent will of his own. The objectionists draw a picture of him in the Caliban image, Prospero's beastlike slave in Shakespeare's *Tempest*, combined with Aldous Huxley's imaginary delta and epsilon. This too will hardly win friends or find acceptance among identical twins or among those who know and love them. And it simply is not true anyway, if that is a consideration in the discussion.

Among those who argue from possible remote consequences there are some who object to cloning because of the unfair and criminal uses it might be put to. This is the wedge argument again. Male chauvinists complain that female chauvinists could use cloning to get rid of men altogether, that they could set up a matriarchy or Amazonia enforced not only by social and political controls but guaranteed biologically.

Another comparable objection is that body cells could be stolen or bootlegged by a cutting stealthily snipped from somebody's arm, so that envious neighbors could gain a genotype which is ours and to which they have no right. We are already familiar with this kind of trickery; it is done all the time, using the ordinary natural mode of reproduction. Perpetrating such tricks by artificial means would in fact be far more complicated and harder to get away with, as well as easier to detect; several medical functionaries would have to be involved.

Comparable psychological objections are raised. Cloning, it is said, could aid and abet an unhealthy narcissism in the kind of people who would want children from their own cells alone. This point, like several other objections, is tied up with the false notion that reproducing from only one genotype results in the same personality profile as the progenitor's. Narcissistic people, self-lovers, simply will not get offspring who are their mere images and mirrors, by cloning.

As for passing on unknown risks, the problem is the same in both sexual and asexual parenting—but *actually less likely in cloning*. To take a hypothetical case, a woman and her husband both carry the gene for a recessive disease; they cannot have a child coitally because it might be defective. She wants to carry her own baby while bypassing the disease, but she does not want to have an insemination from a donor nor to adopt. This being so they could turn to nuclear transplantation. She could have a cell from her own flesh inserted into a denucleated egg and then implanted in her womb. Other times the cell could be the husband's. In this way the fetal combination of their cell nuclei would be avoided, yet each would have a direct descendant.

Personality problems might sometimes provide sound objections to these solutions, but it would be because of the factors in a particular case—unless, as one objector says whole-hog, there is a "right not to be manufactured" which he says ought to rule out the "caprices" of people who would clone their own children.[22]

Virgin Birth Stories

There is, furthermore, a peculiar religious block to be recognized. It arises with pious people when any mention is made of monogenesis—i.e., of virgin birth. They do not like any mention of virgin birth either in its natural forms or when it is induced artificially by cloning. Prospectively there will also be what Rostand once called "solitary generation," i.e., monogenesis by activation of egg or sperm without the manipulation of nuclei required in cloning body cells. It is objected that we are undermining the faith of believers in the Christian doctrine of the Virgin Birth when we point out that virgin birth is not at all unique and when we talk of enacting it at will.†† To the nonpious and non-

---

†† In the underworld of hagiology, the legendry of the saints, Joseph is sometimes regarded as a cuckold, God having pre-empted his husbandly role, evidently without his knowledge and consent. Since God did it by his word, by verbal fiat, they say Mary was "impregnated" through her ear. Nasty little seminarians often speak of the vaginal orifice as the auricula. In Italy, Joseph is referred to as Tio Pepe and appealed to by husbands who suspect they are being betrayed by their wives. See Robertson Davies' *Fifth Business* (Viking Press, 1970, p. 196).

orthodox, on the other hand, this seems to be just one more religious idea that has to be revised or discarded as human knowledge grows, even though so much dogma and controversy and persecution have been invested in it.

This has long been a problem for the traditionalists. It was discussed wisely by a Catholic lay theologian as early as 1931.[23] "Life without father" is no longer supposed to be impossible. In early Christian history Tertullian said he believed in the virgin birth of Jesus because it was absurd, while St. Augustine argued for it on a "natural history" basis—that it happened among animals. Now we know it could happen among humans too.

But it should be noted that a child born of parthenogenesis when it is gynogenic (when it happens to a woman), as in the Virgin and Child story, will always be female. Only male sperm can supply the Y chromosome and without it a normal male is not possible. Yet in the accounts Jesus appears to have been normal, at least in the biological sense. If so, then his birth was not virginal—unless you want to believe he was gestated and delivered without any genes and chromosomes at all. But if he was the child of a virgin birth as the doctrine claims he could not have been a normal man physically. One or the other.

When the Virgin Birth doctrine began to be asserted in the second century A.D. stories were told of "virgin mothers" who had been impregnated from semen in warm bath water first used by a man. The Ebionites, Jews who accepted Jesus as messiah, held that he was born in a fully and directly human way as Joseph's natural son, and like the Ebionites many present-day Christians may go back to the nonvirgin belief of St. Paul, the Mark gospel and the John gospel

—sources of the Jesus story which are entirely without any mention of a "miraculous" birth.

Motherhood in religious mythology has had a changeable place. Among Christians the mother in the Jesus story plays a stellar role whereas in the Creation story there is no mother at all. In Genesis, God was the mother, the first mother. More than that God formed Adam artificially; it was done nonbiologically, with complete artificiality, from the dust. Then Adam in turn became the second mother when Eve was born from his body, his "rib," and God acted as the obstetrician. It was monogenesis all right but not cloning, for had it been cloning Eve would have been a man. Next, Eve was the mother of Cain and Abel‡‡—a female mother at last, on the third round. Women have continued to be the mothers ever since, until now when reproduction once more takes the form of artifice as it did in the Garden of Eden—including motherless children and male mothers.

The Eden myth was that God fixed it for men to reproduce sexlessly or not at all, then the Fall from sinlessness (the snake and apple bit) turned them on to sex, for which he had by his divine foreknowledge prepared them by equipping them with the requisite reproductive apparatus—covered by a fig leaf. Just as Eve was borne by Adam, so we have at last come full circle. The new biology is restoring the non-CG modes which were in effect before the Fall. The difference now is that both the antisexual attitude and the myth are discredited. Sex and reproduction stand on their own merits, no longer tied together.

‡‡ The myth takes a sudden jump from the pangenetic idea that Adam was all mankind's progenitor; Abel is killed by Cain, his only sibling, and then Cain goes off to "the land of Nod" where he finds a wife whose existence is entirely unaccounted for, and unaccountable.

The Debate Gets Rough

Contributory techniques related to the new reproductive medicine also meet lots of objection and opposition. The practice of sacrificing embryos in laboratory fertilization, both in research and in therapeutic procedures such as the Edwards-Steptoe clinic's, is as bitterly denounced as abortion is. Indeed, the two things are equated by some antagonists. One tirade actually spoke of flushing blastocysts away as morally questionable, a hideous practice going on between a "doctor and his plumber." The writer declared that those who terminate pregnancies only look upon a fetus as if it were a "hamburger in the stomach." Language of this kind reveals how deep the feeling runs. It is a kind of semantic assault or what has been called an *"argumentum ad baculinum"*—literally, with a cudgel, striking out in all directions.

When a religious moralist said in a leading medical journal that interruption or termination of a pregnancy is only a euphemism for "killing the fetus" the editor very gently replied that "killing" is just as pejorative or prejudicial as "interruption" is euphemistic.[24] The use of semantic weapons is a debate-stacking device which shows how emotional or wily the antagonists are. Right-to-life propagandists take pains to refer to male and female fetuses as "unborn boy and girl babies" and during a 1972 referendum vote on a more liberal abortion law in a midwest state they had school children call voters on the telephone, saying in a piping youngster's treble, "This is the voice of a little unborn baby."

Closely related to the issue over abortion and the disposal of embryos for research or medical reasons is the new procedure of superovulation. One of its uses is to allow a choice of sex, selecting a male or female embryo and letting the remainder go. In most instances only one or a few of the total number of eggs thus released from an ovary are or would be fertilized, and only part of the fertilized ova (zygotes) are carried forward. The remainder are discarded.

Some sociologists complain that sex selection is unwise because most people would select boys whereas girls read more books, commit fewer crimes, go to more plays, are more religious, and do more about the moral education of children. For some people these value considerations might weigh heavily, but they raise doubts more about our popular values than about either sex selection or superovulation.

It is also charged that if people have enough biological control to choose their children's sex, and if they favor boys in a male chauvinist spirit and a male dominated world, it will throw the sex ratio of the population out of balance. This fear would have made more sense back in the days when *under*-population was the danger, but far fewer females are needed now to keep up the baby supply to a social-survival level. It also presupposes the baby machine image of women, perhaps unconsciously. But as fewer babies are wanted in the new era and the modes of reproduction are varied, women will inevitably find and be granted *personal* status—not maternal.

The New York gynecologist's patient, whose story of repeated pregnancies and abortions to bypass Tay-Sachs disease is told in the preceding chapter, will one day be spared her agonies and the loss of "nascent life" involved. Superfetation will allow genetic testing of a medically contrived multiconception, to select the healthy conceptus and eliminate the diseased ones. The patient's health and peace of mind, the expenses, and the time now lost will all be bypassed.

Fairly outlandish objections, pseudo-consequential in form, are trotted out upon occasion. A sample is the complaint that with superovulation and multi-fertilization, followed by gestation in hostesses or sur-rogates, a couple in their twenties could have all their children at once and then be free of child care by their forties. This might be liberating for the parents, they admit, but they insist it would stunt the children to lose their parents' exclusive attention one by one in their infant years. Other and more bizarre scenarios can be put together, given enough imagination. For example, simultaneous gestations carried out in glass wombs, all in a row on a shelf—when ectogenesis be-comes cheaper than surrogation.

Sperm, ova, and embryo banks will also make selec-tion easier, not only for sex and other traits but in order to protect health and genetic quality. But the specter is raised of commercialization, and of profit-seeking undermining medical and social standards. "Eggs for sale" is a common epithet here. Can such banks get germ cells and embryos that measure up to decent standards? Who will guarantee them? What is to prevent deception or fraud, or even just innocent error? Who will set and enforce standards and proce-dures? What is to prevent the state from making a monopoly of sperm banks, sterilizing all men, and thus gaining complete control of human reproduction? A story goes the rounds about a woman who received an artificial insemination (donor) from a sperm bank, then learned too late that it was a *black* embryo she was carrying, and committed suicide. This canard is told obviously to stop any real thinking on the subject among racists.

Genetic "engineering" gets its full share of "flak," of course. Preconceptive control of the individual's in-heritance or genetic constitution is, after all, the last or maybe we should say the first word in biomedical control. It is radical in the literal meaning of the word, going right to the root of things. As we pointed out earlier, gene control goes deeper than the prenatal and contraconceptive phases of birth technology. This being so, journalistic surveys of the new biology often end by saying that the power to modify heredity, to direct and induce mutations, is as dangerous as the atom bomb, too dangerous to tolerate. We cannot know where it might lead us, they say.

A Sir George Pickering (Oxford Regius Professor of Medicine) can say, "I find this a terrifying prospect, and I am glad I shall be dead . . . before it happens," while a Lord Brain (neurologist) pooh-poohs proposals to put a stop to it by pointing out that if we cannot foretell the consequences of making such discoveries we cannot foretell the consequences of not making them either.[25] In the Soviet Union too there is disagreement. A. Neyfakh of the Institute of the Development of Biology, Soviet Academy of Sciences, urges genetic engineering to undergird higher I.Q.s, but A. Petropavlovsky, another scientist, opposes any such program.[26]

The Nobel laureate George Beadle's opinion is that "Man knows enough but is not wise enough to make man."[27] On the other side N. J. Berrill says, "Sooner or later one human society or another will launch out on this adventure, whether the rest of mankind approves or not. If this happens, and a superior race emerges with greater intelligence and longer lives, how will these people look upon those who are lagging behind? One thing is certain: they, not we, will be the heirs to the future, and they will assume control."[28]

The fear of genetic control runs to anxious prophecies of international and ideological competition, with rival nations trying to "engineer" superior intelligence, manual dexterity, memory capacity, physical strength and size, and other qualities. It is not at all clear why a contest over genetics is so threatening. Competition in science is an old story; we have seen it in space science and technology, for example. Would biological competition be "to the death and without quarter," seeing that space exploration and pollution control on earth have already led to an increase of friendly competition, mutual benefit, and exchange of data? Would something like a Geneva Convention stop it? To make a treaty work could we rely on mutual terrorization, as we do in the Strategic Arms Limitation (SALT) agreement with Russia? How could a ban or moratorium keep its no-no on genetic engineering from ruining therapeutic genetics? Can they be separated?

Much of the high feeling—not to say outright animosity—in the debate about genetics and reproductive medicine comes from expressed or unexpressed religious opinions. Such opinions play an *a priori* or first premise role in the arguments of most objectors. In fact most religious people are shocked when a minority in their own circles do not take the "conscientious objector" pose. One of their spokesmen has referred to "theologians-turned-technocrats" who "fly off into the wild blue yonder of limitless self-modification."[29] Their objections on ethical grounds are based in turn on religious grounds, and by definition all faith assertions are neither verifiable nor falsifiable.* For example, the early-nineteenth-century ob-

---

* What can be proved is not a matter of faith; faith is outside the reach of evidence. It is not that faith is necessarily "blind" to facts, but nothing the believer can *see* can prove anything about his belief one way or the other. To paraphrase an old saying about beauty, the faith is in the eye of the believer. Nonfalsifiable propositions have no place in serious debate, as Karl Popper explains in his *Logic of Scientific Discovery* (London, 1959, p. 40).

jection to abortion was its dangerousness medically, but with the favorable changes in termination methods now achieved that kind of moral objection will be altered. But there is little hope of altering ethical objections based on the religious or metaphysical belief that an embryo is a person. The lack of anything like a litmus paper test for the presence of a *person* in the Fallopian tubes or womb puts such morality outside the pale of empirical data and pragmatic reasoning.

Overlooking his loaded language ("stud farm") and his distortions of the issue ("replacement of the family") the religious objector's position is neatly put by a Catholic writer this way: "The scientific humanist may be as much repelled by the prospect of the replacement of the family by the stud farms of artificial insemination as the Christian, but unlike the latter he has no final argument against it. If the power is there why should it not be used?"[30] His suggestion or implication is that faith in God is "final" in the sense that it overrides any arguments for AI based on the humanist's moral standard, and that the church's teaching has God's backing and God is "final" and that's that.

The big hitch in this is that people who believe in God have different beliefs about the divine will. Jews, Christians, Moslems, Buddhists, and Hindus disagree also within their own religious ranks about the new genetics and baby making. Christians, for example, disagree because they have different beliefs about what is natural and how God is related to nature or what God's will is and how to interpret scriptures. This is true of the other religions too.

To illustrate this diversity, look at the opinion of a Benedictine priest. He writes in *The Catholic Medical Quarterly* that objections to abortion as the killing of a "human" being rest only on unverifiable opinion because there is no evidence or revelation for when the soul enters a conceptus. Therefore, he says, it follows with respect to *in vitro* fertilization that "it is possible only to give *opinions* about its morality," not positive condemnations. He adds that "in many instances in the past two centuries the Church has backed the wrong horse and done herself immense harm by having to climb down: this was true of Darwin and Freud, and it may well be that the future will see a similar situation regarding the Church's attitude to sexual morality, to sterilization and even to abortion . . . So I would say, regarding these in-vitro cultures of human ova, that we should not be too dogmatic and condemn out-of-hand those who are honestly researching into the truth. If we do, we may be backing the wrong horse!"[31]

Historically genetics owes a great deal to priests. A Jesuit, Abbé Lazzaro Spallanzani, first showed in 1776 that animals are made from the germ cells; an Augustinian, Abbé Gregor Mendel, first showed in 1865 that traits are inherited through the germ cells; and another Jesuit, Abbé Frans-Alfons, first showed in this century that "crossing over" between chromosomes is the key to how traits are distributed quantitatively in inheritance sexually.

Catholics are not the only ideological opponents. Some right-wing Protestants are too, and for a long while the Soviet biologists under Lysenko put genetics under a prohibition. But in the words of Bernard D. Davis, bacteriologist at the Harvard Medical School, "Genetics will surely survive the current attacks, just as it survived attacks from the Communist Party in Moscow and from fundamentalists in Tennessee. But meanwhile if we wish to avert the danger of some degree of Lysenkoism in our country we may have to defend vigorously the value of objective and verifiable knowledge, especially when it comes into conflict with political, theological, or sociological dogmas."[32]

Not all opponents of abortion, cloning, and genetic control or birth technology claim religious sanctions. Some simply take their stand on grounds of emotion, of a feeling of revulsion. A woman on a national TV panel said, "I guess it's a gut thing with me. I just don't like it, and arguing back and forth isn't going to change how I feel." This honesty and candor deserves respect from her opponents and supporters alike. She speaks for a certain number of people; how many we do not know.

The fact is that her kind of "gut" opinion is not apt to be much changed by rational discourse. Those who clothe it in argument have to be all the *cleverer* because like the storied Emperor it mustn't be seen to be naked. On the other hand, many religiously motivated opponents of the new medical morality strictly avoid the use of religious rhetoric and use other strategies. In any case we are left with a certain residue of either candid or foxy people who are simply not going to be moved by appeals to reason.

IV

SOME ISSUES

Earlier we remarked that biology can solve our
how-to problems but not our what-to problems.
What we *can* do is a scientific question but what we
think we "ought" to do is a moral question. In his
classic essay on population, *The Tragedy of the Com-
mons*,[1] the California biologist Garrett Hardin pointed
out that some problems have no purely technical solution.

Facts are one thing, values are another. They have
a bearing on each other but in the end certainties, prob-
abilities, or possibilities cannot decide desirabilities.
Facts can only help us define the options open to
choice and preference. Even with biology's discoveries
of what can be done about genetic control and reproduction we still have to form a judgment about what
we want—what we believe is good in the making of
human life and how we ought to go about reaching
the good. *Quality control is a moral problem.*

As soon, however, as we try to make moral judgments about things like artificial insemination and
enovulation or cloning we find there are a number of
issues lurking behind the moral choice problems. Our
value judgments hang in turn on how we think or
what we believe about questions prior to value judgments. These are questions of a philosophical kind

about life, reality, the purpose of human existence, what happiness is.

For example, in trying to decide whether embryologists are right or wrong to dispose of fertilized ova in their experiments we find that the answer hinges on what we decide about the claim that zygotes are human beings. The same issue is at the bottom of the abortion debate. In judging whether cloning is right or wrong we first have to examine the claim that individuals have a right to a unique genotype. We cannot determine the morality of genetic engineering until we decide whether there are any limits on man's right to "manipulate" human life. What we think we may or may not do ethically will depend on *how* we think, incidentally, as well as on what we think. Where we stand on these ethical and "meta-ethical" questions will vary according to whether, for example, we decide them by empirical reasoning or religious faith. And so it goes, for nearly everything.

What has been said up to this point can be boiled down to a few major issues waiting in the wings. Each one of them could be elaborated and has been many times, of course. But for our purposes only the bare bones of these conflicts and tensions will be shown. It is worth doing this way because a lot of the time the real issues at stake get hidden in the very process of trying to dig them out. They get twisted and obscured by our prejudices and the verbal smoke we pour out.

Deciding What Is Right

If we try to cope with the morality of birth technology and genetic engineering by simply applying the right-wrong rules of an inherited and "time tested" value system we will most likely be hung up, unable to make constructive judgments because our evaluations are already determined, preset. There are people who persist in deciding things this way. This means at bottom that they have decided not to decide, and to hand their consciences over to an external authority. The authority may be a moral law like the Ten Commandments or a law maker like the Church, but in either case no responsible judgment is allowed.

As we have already noted, there are in the end only two ways to decide what is right. Either we will obey a rule (or a ruler) of conscience, which is the *a priori* or pre-judiced approach, or we will look as reasonably as we can at the facts and calculate the consequences, the human costs and benefits—the pragmatic way.

An actual case reported illustrates the issue in a very typical and human way. A couple was faced with a decision to abort if an amniocentesis showed a severe genetic defect. The husband said, "I was raised Catholic, and . . . I still feel that way . . . my feelings take me one way and my mind another." He and his wife were ready to terminate the pregnancy if the test was positive. Happily, it was not. The reporter of this case of intrauterine diagnosis remarks, "The moral reasoning of the parents was distinctly along consequentialist lines . . . I interviewed no parents who came at their roles from highly conscious norms or principles about parenthood and unconditioned caring." This is very reassuring about the moral sanity of plain people, which they manage to keep in spite of religious-ecclesiastical pressures.[2]

In the language of logic and cognition theory we might say that rules morality is deductive, situation morality is inductive. To the *a priori* approach the nondogmatic decision maker opposes an *a posteriori* way of deciding what to do—deciding after he weighs the pros and cons rather than before he weighs them. In a sense we may say that following moral rules dispenses with thinking. It asks only what the right rule to follow is, not what good might be gained.

However, once we decide to act in the service of *values* rather than of rules we still find we have to decide what our top value is, our ideal or highest good. This book is, for instance, motivated by human well-being. In this approach what is right will be what is most humane, what is most conducive to human welfare and happiness. It is based on loving concern.[3] The issue is between obedience to abstract principles and service to concrete human needs; one is dogmatic, the other compassionate.

A legalistic moralist with fixed moral OK's and no-no's will, in the words of one of them, "always have in mind the premise that there may be a number of things that might succeed better but would be intrinsically wrong means to adopt," and therefore "he will not begin with the desired end and deduce an obligation from this end." Instead, he declares, "there are a great many actions that would be wrong . . . *no matter what good consequences are expected to follow*" (italics added).[4] This ethics is deductive, drawn from rules of "intrinsic" authority; it is not reasoned inductively from the facts in the interest of human needs.

Perhaps the difference can be illustrated by contrasting Catholic medical societies with evangelical Protestant physicians' groups. The former condemn abortion; the latter say a fetus is "at the least a potential and developing human life" yet they endorse induced abortion for reasons of individual health, family welfare, and social responsibility—according to the actual needs of the particular patient.[5]

The essence of this lurking issue is well put for us by Dr. Anne McLaren, a geneticist in Edinburgh. At a meeting in Washington in 1971 she discussed ethics and reproductive technology and remarked that there are two kinds, "the one emphasizing compassion and consideration for people, the other stressing abstract principle . . ."[6]

Means and Ends

Most of us decide for or against things on the principle of proportionate good. We try to figure out the gains and losses that would follow from one course of action or another and then choose the one that is best, the one that offers the most good. This calculation of consequences is often called a trade-off or cost-benefit analysis. Medicine certainly uses this ethical approach, and it thinks of "good" in terms of human health and well-being. Situations have to be examined and relative choices made. This focus on the situation is "clinical" ethics—its treatment is not prescribed in advance or according to some unexceptionable laws of medical or social care.

For example, the automobile involves fifty thousand deaths and two million casualties every year; no other instrument, not even excepting war's killing, hurts so many of our people. But few of us would sacrifice the good the auto does to avoid the evil, by imposing a blanket prohibition. It is our sense of distributive justice which is at work here. The heart of a responsible ethics is this question: "What, of what can be done, should be done; what of what should be done can we afford; and what of what we can afford are we prepared to pay?"[7]

But how many of us ever stop to see that this means that the end justifies the means? It does. (It does *not* mean, of course, that any end will justify any means, regardless of proportionate good.) If we are morally flexible enough to act on the principle of necessity, subordinating secondary values to primary values, and if we tailor our choices relatively or proportionately, it means that we believe the right thing to do is to put first things first and achieve the most good possible— even though we have to use actions we could not justify in other and different situations. We have already noted this about medicine's *nil nocere*, do no harm. Surgeons hurt the flesh and psychiatrists the feelings, upon occasion. In orthopedics a patient may be urged to put weight painfully on a broken joint, or the joint may even be rebroken. Iodine in the past had to be poured into open wounds, but is no longer necessary. So—"do no harm" means, *Do no harm unless the end justifies the means.*

This makes the folklore saying "The end cannot justify the means" a nonsensical maxim, because we believe that only the end (a proportionate good) makes sense of what we do (the means). A *priori* ethics contends adamantly that the end does *not* justify the means, and it does so because for an *a priorist* or universalizer it is moral rules or laws—such as "It is immoral to conceive by donor insemination"—which justify our choices; not the relative or best possible good but the ethical dogmas. This is literally a pre-judiced ethics; it judges prior to the problem.

Here, then, is another very basic issue affecting our way of dealing with genetics and reproductive medicine. A clear illustration is the prohibition of sterilization by religious authorities. The fact that a couple who have been diagnosed as both heterozygous for Tay-Sachs, so that they would want to be sterilized to keep their love making from ending in the tragedy of fetal disease, would make no difference. In law or legalistic ethics as compared to love or humanistic ethics the sterilization would be wrong no matter what the motive, no matter how much good it would make possible or how much evil it would prevent. A compassionate ethics would put the well-being of the married couple first, not the abstract negative prohibition; compassion would hold that the end justifies the means, and that in any moral calculus human need is the principal value.

We are assuming that people are rational even though we know that they are not wholly so. Our decisions are visceral as well as cerebral. But there is no other model than the rational one on which to base our ethical approach. "Original sin" (the notion that human reason as well as the will to do good is "fallen") was for a long time taken seriously, and there are various other antirational doctrines of a more contemporary kind. By definition they all repudiate any attempt to be ethical because they deny human ability and freedom. So here is yet another basic moral issue: Are human beings hopelessly mired in moral failure, or *can* we achieve a higher level of values and purpose?

Are There Any Human Rights?

At about the time that Shakespeare's *Love's Labour's Lost* appeared, by an ironic coincidence an English surgeon named Peter Chamberlen tried to keep secret his invention of forceps to help delivery in childbirth. He wanted to sell it and make a profit. After all, he was only acting on his "right"—the right of private property, of copyright or intellectual property. But if we have any idea that he was morally wrong we are putting human needs before rights. The whole ethical tradition of medical care and research says that Chamberlen was wrong—that human needs come first, not rights.

All sorts of rights are asserted. They are sometimes even thought to be given in the nature of things ("natural rights"), objectively valid claims which may not morally be denied. At least sixty-three "human rights" are said to be imbedded in the U. S. Constitution and its amendments.[8] Documents like the English and French Declarations of the Rights of Man (1689 and 1789), Tom Paine's *The Rights of Man* (1791–92) and the UN Declaration (1948) and Covenants on Human Rights are among the most glorious of our political-legal achievements.

At the same time, however, serious thinking has always recognized that these rights are "imperfect" or relative; sometimes one or more of them conflicts with others. They cannot therefore be self-validating or absolute or universal. The official report of a presidential commission (1968) on violence in America was entitled *Conflicts in Rights*.

The question arises: When rights are in conflict and one or another supposed right has to be set aside, how do we choose—by what standard or first-order value do we rank them? The answer of course is "the greatest good of the greatest number." Human *need* comes first, and the general welfare or widest need prevails. This principle has been a part of civilization since long before democracy gave it a formal structure or the English utilitarians gave it a popular formula. Typhoid Mary's right to freedom of travel is restricted for the common good.

In the same way other needs, for health for example, come before relatively less urgent rights. The main point to grasp is that human needs validate human rights, not the other way around. The sanction for our humanistic ethics lies in need; need is the court of appeal.

There is no necessity here to catalogue so-called rights. They are all subject to moral weighing; sometimes they pass the critical test of human needs and sometimes they fail it. The "right to life," for instance, is qualified by justifiable homicide. The "right to die" is gaining acceptance as the need for human dignity and compassion in terminal illness is shown more and more urgently with the use of resuscitative medicine and various artificial life-support systems. There is a rising tide of talk about "the right to health" as our need for some kind of national insurance and a more just distribution of medical care eats away at our consciences. The right to have control of one's body has long been recognized in the requirement of the patient's consent to surgery. The same right of self-determination plays a growing role in the abortion debate, in refusals of transfusions and transplants, and in patients' decisions against the prolonging of life medically. The story of human rights shows how they have first been acknowledged under the pressure of human need, and how changed human needs may then suspend or even cancel them later under different conditions. (This last development is by now almost the case with the "right" to bear arms, for example; it is now a right which is no longer right but a limited *privilege*.)

What, then, of the "right to reproduce" and the "right to be born" and even—as a few people have been claiming—the "right to be born with a unique genotype"? Dogmatic moralists will say "A right is a right" and if parents want to reproduce it is their "God-given right." Humanistic or personistic moralists will say, "A right depends on human well-being, and if the parents are both carriers of a recessive gene causing lifelong pain and misery for the child they would have, then they should not conceive—the right is null and void." The right to be parents ceases to run at the point of victimizing the offspring or society.

Dogmatists even claim that embryos or fetuses "have" the right to be born—raising the whole question how it is possible to assign rights to nonpersons. But humanists will say, "No. If a potential baby will be born into tragic subhumanness, and if we know it, we are morally obliged to prevent its birth if we can." Not to stop it in such a situation makes us accessories to a human wrong. There is no such thing as a right knowingly to bring crippled children into the world. And now we *can* know. And as to the alleged right to a unique genotype, far better a cloned child well and strong and fit for life than a deformed or defective child whose genotype happens to be unique.* Opposition to genetic engineering takes the form "We have no right to tinker with human cell nuclei," while the counter opinion is, "Tinker when human happiness needs it." The former is *a priori*, the latter is consequential.

Let's Play God

The Dean of St. Paul's in London once quoted William McDougall: "The great function and tendency of religion, once established among a people, is to preserve intact the current moral code and to se-

---

* Happens is the correct word. So-called unique genotypes are accidents of sexual combination—what we have called reproductive roulette—as compared to the resigned genotypes of genetic engineering and cloning. The fact is, however, that even identical twins with the same genotype may have significant differences, if a mutation occurs in one of the two. They all have different fingerprints, at least. Uniqueness is not so unique.

cure conformity to it."[9] This influence is at work in the complaint that when men try to control their genetic makeup or to start and stop pregnancies they are "playing God"—trying to invade God's privileges and prerogatives. They often tie the charge of ungodliness or impious pride to "interfering with nature." Nature is believed to be God's creation and plan, and therefore an artificial human contrivance is a presumptuous form of playing God, especially if it takes the place of natural modes and processes—for example, coital conception.

Once God was the final court of appeal in morality. That was possible because most social communities shared the same beliefs about God and accepted the same "revelations." All of that is changed; it's over with. Now we live in pluralistic societies with mobile populations; jet travel in the air moves us in a day from one distant culture and religion to another. This makes it impossible to go on thinking about God in the simple consensual way we did when we lived in an isolated, immobile, separated world. Even those who still believe in God realize that they cannot draw universal norms or rules of conduct for daily living and decision making from what they happen to believe about God or the supernatural. More and more, now, believers claim only that God commands us to act lovingly, to be concerned with human need and well-being. *How* to do this is no longer prescribed in codes but open-ended and up to responsible moral agents.

Prescientific, nonrational, "old morality" taboos, with or without claims of divine authority, are going down the drain. Only an ethics rooted in human well-being can or should survive the pressures of man's struggles and advances. Churches will either be transformed along with ethics, or die. Careful thinkers are convinced that religion in the age of science cannot be sustained by the assumption of miraculous events abrogating the order of nature. Instead, we should see acts of God in events the natural causes of which we fully understand. The position now is that men, not God, are the ones who are "abrogating" natural processes.

Fatalism and Control

To say that we cannot or should not treat genetic disorders before or after conception is fatalism. It is an attitude of passive endurance toward life. People still feel that genetic inheritance is blind fate, that we are as foreordained by genes as astrologists say we are by the stars; they insist that the genes cannot or ought not to be altered. Its religious form is "God wills it, and whatever he wills is what must be. So be it. *Selah* and *Amen*." Its nonreligious form is simply put in the familiar song *"Que será, será,"* "Whatever will be, will be."

Any suggestion that moral questions are outside the scope of legitimate human decision is an ethical form of fatalism. This is what *a priori* or dogmatic ethics is. It can say, for example, that laboratory fertilizations or nuclear transplants are immoral and therefore not ever open to human choice and responsibility. In this perspective we must submissively and fatalistically accept the diseases and barren marriages that could sometimes be overcome. Compassion and humanistic ethics, on the contrary, asks for human control over such misfortunes. We might call the issue control ethics versus fatal ethics, or choice ethics versus chance ethics.

To take a very simple illustration, tests of amniotic fluid from a pregnancy are now available to warn of the prospect of respiratory disease, a condition that kills twenty-five thousand infants every year in the

United States. It is fatalism to say as some moralistic people do that we ought to "keep out of the womb." If we believe that the responsible thing is to practice control and try to increase human happiness we are "responsibilists" or "voluntarists." The issue is whether we can and ought to take away the blindfold over our eyes or go on trying to live under the tyranny of the Fates, the three daughters of Darkness. In the Bible's mythology the issue is whether people should disregard Jehovah's prohibition and eat the fruit of the tree of knowledge in Eden; or whether the tower should be built above Babel—that is, stay "humbly" ignorant and helpless or stand up as tall as we can.

Nature-Nurture

Still another way to express the issue between fatalism and moral freedom, or between *a priori* universal negatives and situational discretion (to put it in the language of ethics) is seen in the long-standing nature versus nurture debate. Are we better off going by what nature provides or by nurturing human invention, by trying to improve on nature or taking it as it is?

This is an old issue which has sprung up again fiercely in today's scene in campaigns to protect the environment. In social biology a major and urgent question is how to maintain the ecological balance between civilization and the environment. All signs point to a serious imbalance. "Hardware" technology has been allowed to run wild, putting things out of kilter with its pollution, foolish land use, and the exhaustion of natural resources. In consequence spaceship Earth could conceivably be scuttled.

Some of us tend to turn the problem into a dilemma. Either we embrace what the Germans call Natur-

Mystik and go "back to nature" demanding an end to technology, or we go whole-hog for technology at whatever cost, in a sink-or-swim spirit or with a naïve wish-thinking confidence that technology itself will somehow save us from our excesses: so—eat, drink, and be merry. But this turning the problem into a radical either-or issue, simplistically, dangerously falsifies reality whether we are coping with hard technology and the environment (the biosphere) or with soft technology and reproductive medicine.

René Dubos, whose love and appreciation of nature has distinguished him, recently struck a wise note in the midst of the discord.[10] He flatly rejected the evangelical environmentalists' reactionary posture, for example Barry Commoner's "fourth law of ecology," *nature knows best*. Dubos denied that human interference with nature is *as such* wrong or undesirable. "Only the most starry-eyed Panglossian optimist," he said, "could claim that nature knows best how to achieve population control."

The same rational view applies to human biology. Genotypes do not alone determine what a person is, nor, on the other hand, are interpersonal and social influences the whole story. Making a nature-nurture issue of it, natural processes *or* human control, is a useless and obfuscating way of looking at the problem.

Nevertheless, the issue still remains. Who is to be boss? Human or nonhuman forces? Even granted that people and nature are interdependent, which should have the priority? Humanists will say people should, naturalists will say nature should. We find one biocentric writer who wants to "extend to the whole of the biotic world the Kantian precept that persons must be treated not as means but as ends unto themselves."[11]

But can we? Can we really treat whatever nature offers as equally precious with human persons? Can we simply accept natural sterility in a patient, fore-going any nurture in the form of transplants or clon-ing? What should we do when nature and human needs conflict? Dubos thinks that the biocentric slogan "nature knows best" is a kind of Franciscan irrespon-sibility, compared to the Dominican stewardship in the anthropocentric outlook he himself advocates. Vitalism has too many quandaries.†

Having reverence for life is one thing, making it sacrosanct is another. It is immoral to treat life, just because it is life, as always sacred. *Human* life would be closer to being sacred, but even there we have to compare and choose sometimes.

The upshot is well stated by the immunologist Sir Peter Medawar: "It is a profound truth . . . that na-ture does not know best; that genetical evolution, if we choose to look at it liverishly instead of with fatu-ous good humor, is a story of waste, makeshift, com-promise, and blunder."[12] Jesus talked about bringing a more abundant life—a life of quality, not mere life. Raw nature is often painfully indifferent to human values. It is unmoral.

Yet to mention values and to speak of "quality of life," the QOL of so much ecological and biomedical discussion, obviously presupposes an anthropocentric or human-oriented outlook. Values are values for *peo-ple*. To be biocentric or nature-oriented is, like na-

† In its ethical meaning vitalism is the doctrine that life is the highest good—higher than personal values. It leads to a refusal, for example, to let a hopelessly dying patient go as long as his or her biological functions can be dragged on by natural or artifi-cial means. It demands that a severely deformed newborn (per-haps a case of radical spina bifida) should nonetheless be res-pirated and "saved" for a few years of heightening pain and dehumanization. (There is a cosmological meaning for vitalism too: the belief that physics and chemistry cannot account for biological life, that an *élan vital* of some kind is behind or beneath it.)

ture, to have no interest in values or quality. Nature's drive is only for survival, by means of quantity, not quality, in order to compensate for its waste—like using hundreds of millions of spermatozoa to fertilize one human egg, and equipping girls with a half million egg cells (oöcytes) when only five hundred will ever be released and no more than a maximum of forty could possibly be gestated.

As a matter of fact the term "nature" has a multitude of meanings, and therefore none practically. Webster's gives thirteen synonyms: essence, creation, constitution, structure, disposition, truth, regularity, kind, sort, character, species, affection, and naturalness. Except for species, and maybe constitution and structure, every one of these words is question-begging. The dictionary also offers eleven different definitions. The best one, least subject to misunderstanding or semantic tricks, is "the sum total of things in time and space; the entire physical universe." This means that laboratory fertilizations, cloning, and glass wombs are as natural as love, life and death, and the sunset. Bottle feeding of babies may often be less desirable than breast feeding but it is not because bottle feeding is "unnatural"—even though some say it is, as they also said about anesthesia when it was first used in childbirth.

Humanness and Abortion

For some of us "human nature" is fixed, a given entity; for others the human organism and psyche are malleable and adaptable. T. E. Hulme said, "Man is an extraordinarily fixed and limited animal whose nature is absolutely constant."[13] To the contrary Ashley

Montagu explains that babies are not born with a human nature, only with more or less capability of *becoming* human.[14] In the same vein the Spanish philosopher Ortega y Gasset concluded that people have no nature; they have only their histories.[15]

When Montagu speaks of babies "becoming human" what does he mean? What does it mean to be human; what exactly *is* a "human being"? Have we an inventory of its traits—a humanhood agenda? This is a crucial question because so many ethical problems hang on it; different opinions about humanness will result in different moral decisions. Philosophers and theologians in the past have spoken very smoothly about the *humanum* but their abstract and metaphysical rhetoric never got down to a biological approach, which might yield more helpful specifics and a more meaningful definition.

Actually, we have to ask whether it is human life we put first or *personal* life? If it is personal human life, then our first-order concern is with certain qualities and capacities, not just human life as such. In short, may we use "a human life" and "a person" interchangeably? The philosopher Henry David Aiken calls it "fetishism" to believe that a fetus is already a person. But is he justified in saying so?[16] This question is of the greatest practical importance in making decisions about such matters as the terminally ill and when to let the patient go, in dealing with irreversible coma, and whether we ought to "save" what are called monsters at birth. When we quote the Socratic maxim Know Thyself, what *is* the self, the person? Not to know what we mean by these key terms is simply to flounder around when we talk about moral decisions.

Abortion provides a test. Ethically the core issue is whether an embryo or fetus is a human being, and if so in what sense we call it that. How we assess the morality of abortion follows from how we answer this question.

For example, a Catholic lawyer says flatly, "One person's freedom to obtain an abortion is the denial of another person's right to live."[17] He believes that a fetus is a person or has a person's rights. There is no argument, of course, about a human fetus being a stage of the species *homo sapiens*; it is easily recognizable biologically. Nor is there any question of its being alive. Cell division is proceeding. But what about claims of personhood or humanhood for a fetus? If every human fetal organism is a person, and if we think it is immoral to end such forms of human life unnecessarily—at least when self-defense or the common security is not at stake—we will logically look upon abortion at will as immoral. If, on the other hand, we do not regard uterine life as human in the sense of a personal being we will not believe its termination is "murder"—that is, we won't see it as taking the life of an innocent person. The nonpersonal view of fetuses fits in with the morality of elective abortion or abortion on request, as well as with therapeutic abortion for medical reasons.

The ethical issue is dramatized in a mind-blowing situation in a Nazi concentration camp.[18] A Romanian woman doctor secretly aborted three thousand Jewish women in the camp because if they were pregnant on medical report they would be incinerated—sent to the ovens. If we believe that a fetus is a person it would follow that the doctor by killing three thousand human beings saved three thousand others and prevented the murder of all six thousand. On the nonpersonal basis we would say only and quite calmly that three thousand persons were rescued from a terrible death. (The U. S. Congress agreed with the latter interpretation.

She was admitted to residence and citizenship in America as a war hero.)

The most basic issue is whether a fetus is a person or not. This in turn poses the question, "What's the *essence* of a person?" Along with it goes the related question, "When does this essential element emerge, whatever it is?" The question what a person is hinges on whatever is held to be the essence. There would be room for some variety of opinion on additional factors, the other things which make for the fullness or optimum of a person. The decisive problem is to identify the essential thing, the *sine qua non*, that without which there is no person. And to find this key is to get pretty close to answering the question about "when" a person is.

What are the factors or components which people have suggested is the essential one? There are three of them, basically. Some argue that life is the essential element in a person's being; whenever and as long as we are alive, as long as life is present, they say, a human organism is a person. This would mean that a person exists at fertilization when life gets started, and continues to exist through the whole complex biological continuum. Indeed, *before* fertilization oöcytes and sperm are "alive." Death is not complete until the cessation not only of bodily functions but even of cell activity. This opinion identifies the person with life, making the two coexistent or even one and the same. It is the doctrine behind recent agitation to prohibit tests and research with live abortuses, even though there is no possibility of the fetus surviving and even though the knowledge to be gained by obstetricians and pediatricians could save the lives or health of many children yet to be born. It is a radical and sad consequence of an absolute sanctity-of-life ethics.

A second notion is that not life but the soul makes

a person. In this camp we find two different ideas about the soul's entrance into the living tissue. While they both agree that it enters somehow before the birth of the individual, some guess or believe that the soul or *animus* enters after conception, probably in the second trimester ("delayed animation") and others guess it enters with fertilization ("immediate animation")—thus coinciding, in the latter case, with the *life* theory. An obvious absurdity of this latter doctrine is that it means the soul or person of identical twins has been split in two, since after fertilization they separated from a common cell mass or single fertilized ovum. Triplets, quadruplets, and so on, add to the absurdity of the ensoulment-at-fertilization doctrine. Aristotle, Augustine, and Aquinas held to the late ensoulment theory and therefore justified abortion at least in the first trimester; Tertullian, the great heretic, declared for the fertilization idea and his opinion finally became the official Catholic teaching in 1869, when abortion was condemned at any stage. (The papacy has never actually said when the soul is infused; rather, it has decreed that people must play it safe by acting *as if* the soul was infused at fertilization.)

The third opinion is that the essence of a person is reason, the rational function, the *ratio*. On this view everything depends on the mental capability of the individual. This is not to say that reason is everything; feeling is an important part of mental function too. But without intelligence the feeling alone is subhuman. The cerebral has to undergird the visceral. Before cerebration comes into play, or when it is ended, in the absence of the synthesizing or *thinking* function of the cerebral cortex, the person is nonexistent—or, put another way, the life which is functioning biologically is a nonperson. This nonpersonal condition can be seen both in the protoplasm at the start of life and in the "human vegetable" which is sometimes all that remains at the end.

Humans without some minimum of intelligence or mental capacity are not persons, no matter how many of their organs are active, no matter how spontaneous their living processes are. If the cerebrum is gone, due to disease or accident, and only the midbrain or brainstem is keeping "autonomic" functions going, they are only objects, not subjects—they are its, not thous. Just because heart, lungs, and the neurologic and vascular systems persist we cannot say a *person* exists. Noncerebral organisms are not personal.‡ According to this third view perhaps something like a score of 20 on the Binet scale of I.Q. would be roughly but realistically a minimum or base line for personal status. Obviously a fetus cannot meet this test, no matter what its stage of growth.

Nor can a fetus have any of the other traits that make for the full *humanum* or personal quality, such as curiosity, affection, self awareness and self-control, memory, purpose, conscience none of the distinctive transbiological indicators of personality. The fetus-is-a-person doctrine is of necessity the most argumentative one because it has to defend an arbitrary assertion. The nonpersonal view is under no such strain. It asserts nothing not in evidence, and therefore it

‡ The Harvard Medical School's *ad hoc* committee accepted the "brain death" definition but it is too undiscriminating. So is the Kansas statute modeled on it, and the recent (1972) ruling of the Italian Council of Ministers. It is not the death of the *brain* that counts. What is definitive is the absence of cerebration or "mind" even though other brain functions continue. A "human vegetable" is not a person, not truly a human being. It goes without saying, of course, that the loss of the cerebral function must be determined to be irreversible.

really does not have to be defended or make a case for itself.

Antiabortion agitators often say, "Well, anyway, there is a *potential* in the fetus for all of these things that make up a person; for example, the morphon or rudimentary physical basis of mind is present by the eighth month." This is tantamount to admitting that a fetus is in fact not a person. And to argue (which is what this is—*arguing*) that the potential is the actual is like saying that an acorn is an oak or a promise is its fulfillment or a blueprint is a house. The "as if" argument is a prolepsis which tries to wipe out the vital difference between what is and what could be. Thomas Aquinas was at least right to distinguish between human life *in potentia* and *in sit* (actual) and to assign personal status only to the latter, after several months' gestation.

The plain inescapable fact, as a chemist might say, is that we have no litmus paper test for the presence of a person. Jean Rostand, the French biologist, puts it this way: "It must be said that these differing opinions are held by people who are equally sincere, have the same level of morality, and sometimes even profess comparable philosophical doctrines."[19] Any attempt to impose one "doctrine" on others who do not share it is ethically intolerable. We are driven to admit that if anybody wants to believe a fetus is a person at conception or whenever it is "ensouled" he is entitled to. It is a kind of mental Mexican stand-off.

The only possible moral test of these rival views lies in their consequences. When beliefs or nonempirical opinions, neither of them being falsifiable, contradict or clash with each other, the only possible way to choose between them morally is in terms of their consequences if they are followed out logically in practice. The one which results in greater good for people is the correct one. On this basis there is an open and shut case for abortion, obvious and overwhelming; it can be justified very often, sometimes for reasons of human health, sometimes for reasons of human happiness.

Furthermore, the question of *when* the person comes into existence, the timing, has never found any general agreement or any convincing evidence favoring one opinion over others. In the past people have argued variously that this event or "moment" is at (1) fertilization, (2) the blastocyst or implantation stage, (3) the first heartbeat, (4) the phenomenon of "kicking" or "quickening," (6) viability—when the fetus might maintain its life outside the womb (sometime in the third trimester), and finally (7) birth. Here too we have no litmus paper test, no diagnostic criteria. When the Grand Mufti of Jerusalem says the "moment" is the 120th day of pregnancy, like the theologians who used to say it was forty days in the case of males and eighty days for females, we can only try to keep a straight face.

The most sensible opinion is Plato's, that a fetus becomes a person at birth—after it is expelled or drawn from the womb, its umbilical cord cut, and its lungs start to work. This has been the opinion held down through the centuries in the common law tradition. It was not until the nineteenth century that abortion was for the first time made a crime—although, be it noted, only against the state because of the supposed loss of a much needed citizen, soldier, or worker. Crowded subways and expressways, growing lists of hard-core unemployment in the midst of highly productive industrial and agricultural machinery—these things make the "public interest" of a century ago archaic.

Later on, some groups began to claim that abortion

is a crime against the *fetus* as well as against the state, with the result in America that new laws began to prohibit termination of pregnancy for any reason other than to save the woman's life or, in a few states, her health. In spite of these new statutes, however, no prosecutor has ever returned an indictment for murder in any abortion case before the courts. In cases of miscarriage no birth certificates are made out and abortions of such fetal tissue are not entered into the vital statistics. Pregnant women traveling abroad have not been required to carry two passports, one for themselves and one for the fetus. Miscarried embryos at a primitive stage are not baptized.

On and on we could go, pointing out similar lapses or discrepancies between what people preach and what they practice. In 1972, before the Supreme Court's decision in January 1973, spokesmen for the Right to Life Movement carried around a fairly fully formed human organism, superficially, and displayed it for the shock effects on uncritical and impressionable people in audiences. When they were asked if the fetus had been baptized or entered into the birth statistics, christened with a name, and "Why hasn't this child, as you call it, been buried with respect?"—only mumbles, not even clear words, could be heard.

For some time legislators and courts have been revamping those Victorian laws in a return to the main tradition, to the view that a fetus is not a person or what American lawyers call a "Fourteenth Amendment person." The chief reason for the postnatal definition of a person in the law is that any other doctrine is necessarily only a matter of private faith or belief, and it is morally unjust to impose private beliefs upon others who do not share them. To do so violates the First Amendment of the Constitution which guarantees religious freedom and freedom of thought.

The U. S. Supreme Court on January 22, 1973, declared that it is unconstitutional for any state to forbid abortion in the first trimester, which only reaffirms the historic position of Western civilization.** The question *when* a pregnancy should be terminated for health reasons is a medical one, the Court explained, and not a proper government function.

In any case, in the last resort it remains the patient's choice, on the principle of consent, as in any other medical or surgical treatment. This freedom of choice coerces no physician into doing an abortion nor any patient into having one. The Court did not enter into the ethical-moral question, it is true, yet by finding for the nonpersonal view of fetal life it put the focus where it really belongs and more profoundly affected the moral issue than any court judgment for hundreds of years.

Only if we can decide where we stand on these issues can we decide where we stand on the morality of terminating pregnancies. In practical policy terms there are four positions to choose among, and our choice will depend on what we decide about the status and quality of the fetus. (1) We can condemn abortion altogether, or at most only justify it to save the pregnant woman's life. (2) We can favor a limited permissiveness to prevent ill health, to prevent defective babies, or to prevent the product of rape or incest. This is a policy of compulsory pregnancy but with escape clauses. (3) We can approve of abortion for any

** This decision knocked down restrictive statutes in forty-six of the fifty states of the Union. It means that freedom of abortion may not be regulated in the first six or seven months—and even then, after the first six months, it would only be *allowed* to the states, not required. The Court rejected any assignment of *personal* status to the fetus at any stage, and allowed only that a government might find a public interest in *potential* human life, and even then not until the fetus has become capable of survival independently of the maternal body. It has no rights.

reason prior to viability—possibly on the ground of social needs or some question of justice, although these grounds are not so apparent as they were when we lacked enough labor power and needed lots of soldiers. (4) We can oppose any and all forms of compulsory pregnancy, making the ending of pregnancies, like their beginning, a private or personal matter.

If we adopt the sensible view that a fetus is not a person there is only one reasonable policy, and that is to put an end to compulsory pregnancy. The ethical principle is that pregnancy when wanted is a healthy process, *pregnancy when not wanted is a disease*—in fact, a venereal disease. The truly ethical question is not whether we can justify abortion but whether we can justify compulsory pregnancy. If our ethics is of the humane brand we will agree that we cannot justify it, and would not want to.

Many sensitive people who support abortion in principle nevertheless see it as a sad, even tragic, action. In this view abortion is a reason for regret, but not for remorse or moral guilt. To deplore abortion is *a fortiori* a strong reason to advocate contraception. To condemn both—both the termination and the *prevention* of unwanted pregnancies—is an antisexual and inhumane morality. (This is what the official Catholic teaching does, except that it allows "natural" birth control by "rhythm," and it helps us to understand the grass roots revolt of Catholics who defy the ban on both contraceptives and sterilizations.)

Process, Not Event

Another basic issue is raised between those who look at life phenomena episodically and those who

view them epigenetically. This is a big-word way of
saying that the question is: Is human life an event or
a process? Or death, for that matter. Is the fetus, for
example, a pattern or chain of incidents (fertilization,
implantation, viability, and so on) or is it a pattern of
development on a continuum? As Cyril Means has
remarked, a live human sperm and egg exist *before*
fertilization; all that occurs is that two squads of
twenty-three chromosomes each form up a platoon of
forty-six, but "there is no more human life . . . than
there was before."[20] In human reproduction, the point
is, life never begins—it is only passed on by means of
conception. Biology shows us that the process principle
is the right one.

Even fertilization is a process—it takes at least two
hours to complete the union of sperm and ovum. We
simply cannot speak of the "moment" when life or
death or mind or anything else biotic "occurs." They
are not occurrences. All talk about a "human being"
occurring at "the moment of conception" is old wives'
talk. It is possible, presumably, to simply assert that
the "soul" is "infused" at some point into a fetus in a
single moment, but this is because there is no possible
way to check it out. Nobody has ever seen one.

A person or personality is certainly not merely a
quick event or episode. It takes many years to assemble
a personality. A newborn baby starts excitingly soon
to take on and store away the makings of a person, but
even so it takes a long time. It is a process that starts
at birth with whatever genetic constitution it has been
physically formed by but it takes a considerable continuum to show results. Even the "switchboard" of the
cerebral cortex needs several years of infancy and child-
hood to get the "wires" of the nervous system and
brain "hooked up" for adequate human performance
and growing up.

What Is Authentic Relationship?

Rostand puts the quality of personality succinctly: he says first, "There is a constant interaction between the physical person and the moral person," but he then adds that "the psychic must be given the priority over the corporal"—meaning the moral is more basic than the physical.[21]

The same thing exactly should be said about *relationship*, about the interpersonal side of our lives. The bonds which tie people together are moral, mental, emotional—not biological. Parents, siblings, and kinsfolk are no "closer" to us than our spouses, friends, neighbors, and fellow men in general. What constitutes a genuine relationship is shared caring and concern, not "blood" or genes or genital origin. By definition friends and lovers cannot be indifferent to each other, but cousins can. Sometimes even siblings and parents are, if they are not actually inimical. The saying "Blood is thicker than water" is on very shaky legs, and the less primitive societies are, the thinner the blood gets.

In an adoption the true father is the one who loves and rears the child, not the one who merely sired it, and the same goes for the mother as distinguished from the gestator. There is no moral reason to hide adoption; the Japanese are rightly proud of adoptee and adopter alike. The legal tradition in the old days was always explicitly "physicalist" about relationship, for example in deciding "rights" of inheritance by "blood" (genes) or consanguinity. Only in recent years have the courts begun slowly to give the possession of children to those who deserve them rather than to those who could establish biological kinship. This gives it *moral* validity; parenthood is not determined solely by a physical fact.

This has been the view of the courts increasingly in adoption contests. In divorce cases when the wife seeks sole custody of a child conceived by A.I.D., but with the husband's consent, the courts have upheld the husband's claims as equal with the wife's. Again in Rostand's words, "since law, morality, and humanism demand that the notion of the person be saved, it is indispensable to dissociate it from the notion of the body."[22]

Artificial insemination and enovulation, along with hostess and artificial gestation, are like adoption, deepening our perception of what family relationship is. Ectogenesis in the broadest sense, not only of being grown outside the womb but also of being conceived apart from the genital intercourse and even the genes of one's parents, yet for all that truly related to those who chose it this way, still a real family—this is a revolution in ethics of the profoundest order.

The thought that a child can be mine even though not "the seed of my loins" is not altogether new. Remember what Sarah said to her husband Abraham when she was sure she could not conceive. "I pray thee go in unto my maid; it may be that *I* may obtain children *by her*" (Genesis 16:12). The child would be Sarah's even though it came by means of her maid's body and not by hers. Now with artificial insemination Sarah no longer needs to ask her husband to engage in adultery, but the principle is the same. And with cloning either Sarah or Abraham could have a child without having to depend on the other, even though they are "too old," and have no need to depend on a miracle any more. And with glass wombs any further need to drag the maid into it to carry the baby to term could be bypassed.

These new methods of reproduction have in concept outmoded the old morals of family relationship and opened up a whole new understanding of relationship. As Jesus said in a challenge to the nonmoral and purely materialistic idea of family, "Who is my mother? and who are my brethren? and he stretched forth his hand toward his disciples and said, Behold, my mother and my brethren!" This moral understanding of family membership goes not only for adopted children but for those procreated by artificial insemination, egg transfers, gonadal transplants, clonings—all reproductive and genetic engineering.[23]

How we understand relationship will have its consequences. It will color and shape our moral judgments about such questions as "Is A.I.D. adultery and the child a bastard?" and "Is a child born of laboratory fertilization an orphan or unparented?" and "Is a baby conceived from an ovary or testicle transplant the donor's child?" and "Is a cloned child thereby denied all family ties?" and "Does genetic intervention cancel or compromise a child's descendancy?" What do we think it really means to belong to a family? What, in fine, constitutes authentic relationship?

With all of these background issues in mind we are ready at last to take a sharp close look at the moral choices we are going to have to make, sooner or later, about the new genetic controls and birth technologies.

V

SOME ANSWERS

When we discuss issues calling for more than a merely technical solution the effect can be much like a centrifuge. We whirl the things we wonder about around and around and the answers finally take shape. They make their appearance by their own weight. Here, then, are a couple of dozen such answers to questions; questions about what is good and what is evil in the new biology and medicine, or what has been called bioengineering.

As we have seen, these answers are based upon a humane concern for the well-being of people, according to actual needs in actual situations. They do not rest on religious doctrines or metaphysical ideas, nor on the prejudicial notion that we ought to follow moral rules regardless of cases or consequences. The "God Squad" approach is too inflexible to fit the variety of real-life situations. In other words, we do not suppose that what is right or wrong can be settled dogmatically in advance of the facts.

Sometimes abortion would be right, sometimes wrong; sometimes egg transfers would be a good thing, sometimes not. The same thing holds true with test tube conceptions, sterilizations, artificial gestations, preselection of sex, cloning, insemination and enovulation from storage banks, and so on. This is the "clinical" approach typical of biomedical ethics.

The main guidelines we have established are these six: compassion, consideration of consequences, proportionate good, the priority of actual needs over the ideal or the potential, a desire to enlarge choice and cut down on chance, and a courageous acceptance of our responsibility to make decisions. With these principles we can arrive at some reasonable conclusions about the morality of human reproduction and genetics.

For convenience's sake the answers are laid out by title in alphabetical order; it will be obvious that a good deal of cross-reference and blending ("interface") develops between many of them—a kind of moral fabric.

Adultery

The traditional literary sense of "adultery," as an interpersonal and intergenital affair, is the correct one. Properly understood, adultery is *only* a personal and genital act. No longer can we say that a monogamous marriage agreement means exclusive access to any or all of the wife's or husband's "generative" faculties. It might exclude third-party genitalia but not third-party sperm and ova, nor graft gonads which can overcome childlessness and barren marriages. It is morally absurd if the law allows, even only by implication, that a donor of seeds could be named a correspondent in a divorce action.

The law will slowly catch up with humanitarian medicine. Donors of sperm and ova, as such, are *not* adulterers in any ethical sense; they are far less adulterers than the Old Testament "levirate" men who impregnated their dead brothers' childless widows for the sake of their brothers' posterity. Their good deeds were intimately intergenital—which is not true of

donors. Adultery cannot apply any longer to the
donation of the powers of our "loins" to persons in
need just because they are not one's spouse.

Artificial Germination

Inseminating and enovulating artificially stand together, ethically. They are ways of conceiving when
other and more familiar methods cannot work. The
opinion that these procedures are wrong, promulgated
officially by the Catholics and backed by a few Protestants and Jews, rests on two assertions: one is that conception by artificial means is immoral because to be
ethical conception "must" be accomplished by intercourse, and the other is that donating and accepting
sperm and ova between the unmarried is adultery. It is
this dogmatic objection which we are rejecting.

Some people find artificial insemination distasteful
or esthetically objectionable, but they do not brand it
as unethical. They do not try to stigmatize the assist-
ing physician as an accessory to a crime or a "sin." It is
simply ridiculous to argue that a consenting husband
in "AID" makes himself a party to an immoral and
criminal conspiracy. Oklahoma's law giving it legal
status and protecting children so conceived is a precedent for similar laws elsewhere. To say, however, that
the practice is not wrong in and of itself does not mean
it is *always* the right thing to do—as we saw in Ann
Landers' case in chapter III. There are still problems
of when and how it should be done. If the benefits are
too meager or the foreseeable consequences too onerous for parents, donors, or children, it is wrong in those
particular cases.

Artificial insemination from a donor is often in order
when the husband is azoospermic or has a low sperm

count. Premature ejaculation, malformation, and psychological hang-ups are other reasons. It is both silly and sad when people are mired down in a physical rather than a moral notion of true family relationship. Out of this error comes the practice of mixing the husband's ineffective semen with the donor's, so that the husband can be regarded as the "putative" father—a pathetic legal fiction. Most happily of all, we can see in artificial insemination and enovulation from donors a means at last whereby we can have children and still avoid crippling or killing them with our known inheritable defects or diseases.

The glaring fault in our practice of assisted conception, up to the present, has been its secrecy. It is wrong to keep the truth not only from the public but also from the child. This used to be done in adoptions until experience began to discourage it. Deception undermines family relationships psychologically, as well as courting the shock of disclosure or discovery. A brother and sister innocently married some years ago in England, having been adopted when they were infants by different families and renamed; only then did they learn the truth, by a fluke. Insemination and enovulation from donors should be matters of agreement with the husband, and a formal record made.

To receive an egg or sperm without the spouse's knowledge and consent would be an odd business, hard to justify. It should be recorded officially by the physician along with his notes of serological tests (e.g., venereal disease and the Rh factor), with proper dates, just as in any other medical service. A child could be wrecked emotionally if he found it out without any preparation; an angry spouse or confidant could disclose it for revenge; "rich uncles" could claim criminal conspiracy if they settled money on such children in ignorance of the truth.

In states where the law does not yet protect the rights of "AID" children it should be revealed in order to adopt them, thus securing their status. (What an irony it is that a child who is at least one-half the biological descendant of his parents has less standing in most states than an adopted child who is altogether unrelated biologically.)

Birth Control

As we have seen, birth control covers a great many things besides contraception. Contraconception, a wider category, includes sterilization, whether by chemical, biological, or surgical means. And literally, the control of *birth* as distinct from conception prevention lies in genetic and fetological interventions. The key to the morality of control is that it should be consistent and complete, not half-baked.

Our moral obligation is to control the quality as well as the quantity of the children we bring into the world. We owe it to a prospective child, to ourselves as parents of integrity, to our families which have only so much in the way of human and economic resources, and to society. Ethically it is in the discretion of a woman to prevent or end any pregnancy she does not want, unless she has promised the child to a husband or lover who justifiably insists on it, or unless a clear case can be made that society has a supervening interest in its birth. (Rarely indeed would either of these limitations cut into her personal freedom.)

Morally this biological self-determination extends as much to legally minor females as to an adult; hence the rapid increase of Minor Consent laws which protect their rights to obstetrical care in spite of obstruction by parents or others.

The looming moral issue has to do with *compulsory* birth control. Up to the present we have relied upon a voluntary policy, and everything else being equal it is better to be responsible for our reproduction of our own free will than to be compelled to. But the two control goals, quality and quantity, cannot rightly be ignored by individuals to the common hurt. Birth control is not merely a private matter. We may have to face compulsory controls of fertility and dysgenic inheritances, however regrettably, as we have had to face compulsory vaccination for communicable diseases.

A contemporary and morally responsible ethics of reproduction calls for whatever policy works. An English clergyman, typifying a not uncommon and truly nihilistic irresponsibility, said recently that without a free private option to reproduce we lose our humanity, and that if therefore population reaches disastrous proportions, "well, then we die."[1]

Laissez-faire has not proved to be altogether a just policy in the production of economic goods and services, Adam Smith to the contrary notwithstanding, and the same can be said of human reproduction. Fortunately, birth control is spreading through all the world, including Asia and Africa, in spite of various religions and customs. We ought not to forget that the original Latin for population, *populare*, meant to devastate or lay waste; it can come exactly to that.

Birth Defects

Children born with defects become at once objects of loving concern. We must do what we can for them, and in some cases *much* can be done. Sometimes, however, voluntary societies seeking help for the mentally "handicapped" or retarded, for the victims of muscular dystrophy, cystic fibrosis, even spina bifida, are—to say the least—sentimental. As much as possible such misery should be *prevented*, not ameliorated. Morally, honest concern for such unfortunate creatures should be based as much on an effort to prevent their birth as to help them when they are born anyway.

Many people plead loud and long for the means to help them, yet they oppose preventive measures such as genetic screening, therapeutic abortion (or embryotomy), gene engineering, artificial germination, sterilization, and most if not all of the reproductive technology which could avoid these tragedies. This is a strange and contradictory species of compassion; it shows up as absurd or phony.

For example, a few die-hard extremists say, "We may not abort defective fetuses; we should work instead on finding cures for genetic and congenital disorders." This is a false either-or, a red herring. Study of abortuses is what gives us the knowledge to eliminate and alleviate these ills. There are those who denounce even embryological studies of blastocysts and primitive embryos; this is a particularly bizarre instance of false compassion.

As it is, obstetricians and pediatricians are put unnecessarily and often in an intolerable quandary. They have to stretch the truth, telling a woman her baby was "stillborn" when it wasn't, after having simply not respirated the delivered fetus—out of mercy for her and her family. If such creatures manage to be born anyway (start breathing) physicians may then resort to high-risk surgery with the unspoken hope that it will be fatal, or they may hold back on antibiotics, a lethal tactic. When these maneuvers fail they then advise putting seriously defective infants in institutions which are nothing more than "warehouses." This is more nearly immoral than moral; it could be escaped as a quandary if our reproductive ethics was honestly based on compassion.

Cloning

Good reasons in general for cloning are that it avoids genetic diseases, bypasses sterility, predetermines an individual's gender, and preserves family likenesses. It wastes time to argue over whether we should do it or not; the real moral question is when and why.

By cloning from the same source, perhaps to preserve biological qualities, clonants would be able to be lifesaving donors to each other of paired or cadaver organs with no risk of failure due to the rejection of alien tissue; this is true already in the case of monozygotic or identical twins. (When an immunosuppressive is found, for what Rostand calls "biological xenophobia," this particular reason for cloning will have lost its weight.) Clonants could always marry nonclonants if they chose to (at the price of thinning out the clone's qualities) but staying strictly within the clone's genotype would be necessary to be sure of nonrejection in transplant operations.

Robert Sinsheimer has remarked that cloning will "permit the preservation and perpetuation of the finest genotypes that arise in our species—just as the invention of writing has enabled us to preserve the fruits of their life work."[2] There could be many other personal and clinical reasons for it in particular cases.

There could also be reasons of the social good. Individuals might need to be selectively reproduced by cloning because of their special resistance to radiation, their small body size and weight, because they are impervious to high-decibel sound waves; these things could be invaluable for professional flights at high altitudes and space travel, for example. In a stretch of imagination, a biologist could solve the weight problem by going alone to a distant planet with a supply of different somatic cells, and colonize it from a cloning start. Even without any need to specialize people we might some day have to turn to either cloning or genetic engineering to correct for the loss of quality we suffer as our recessive defects get spread around in our common gene pool. Dangerous roles within society or on its frontiers might justify cloning, to safeguard those who take risks in the social interest.

What cloning's constructive uses will be cannot, of course, be wholly predicted or even anticipated. Some things can be ruled out. For example, it would be wrong of lesbian or male homophile extremists to want to use cloning to reproduce a general population of their own sex (the males would need at least a few captive ovulators); the fault with it, obviously, would be the loss of genetic variety due to asexual reproduction on such a wide scale, and its undermining effect on the survival of the species.

Inhumane, inordinate suggestions have been made to use cloning to produce legless people, dwarfs, individuals distorted functionally in various ways—for example, to man spaceships to Jupiter. But this seems impossible to justify, given our present knowledge, and would accordingly be morally wrong. Similar is a proposal to solve the fruit picking problem in a future leisure society by using a genetically "designed" and then cloned submental people with prehensile tails to do the work. It can be countered immediately with, "Why not monkeys?" (which are already being considered for some orchards).

There is no ethical objection to cloning when it is

morally (that is, humanely) employed. Artificial virgin births and cloned "multiplets" promise real benefits not only to human beings but to the "green revolution" also. Whole orange groves are sometimes copied tree by tree, from a single high yield tree. Herds of meat and coat animals cloned from a champion Kenya or Kazakhstan sheep could increase our meat supply two or three times in just a couple of years. Fish farming in controlled waters is another option; we need not rely altogether on delicate eco-balances. What men can do by cloning with their plants and animals they could and sometimes should do for themselves. There is no moral reason why we must follow biological heterogeneity in all human beings, whenever homogeneity can serve a constructive purpose.

Control for Quality

An editorial by Dr. Malcolm Watts in the journal of the California Medical Association in 1970 remarked that "man exercises ever more certain and effective control" over the quality of human life. "It will become necessary and acceptable to place relative rather than absolute values on such things as human lives, the use of scarce resources, and the various elements which are to make up the quality of life or of living which is to be sought."[3] All of this, he said, requires "a new ethic" in "a rational development" of "what is almost certain to be a biologically oriented world society."

Physicians in the past, the editorial points out, have tried "to preserve, protect, repair, prolong, and enhance every human life which comes under their surveillance." This was the old vitalistic, undiscriminating sanctity-or-quantity-of-life ethics, now giving way to a responsible, decisional quality-of-life ethics. To repair and prolong lives, indiscriminately, may be a kind of technical virtuosity but it is not *control*. To control means to choose, and therefore any absolute morality about always keeping life going, before or after birth, regardless of quality considerations, is the very opposite of control and a denial of quality.

If we choose family size we should choose family health. This is what the controls of reproductive medicine make possible. Public health and sanitation have greatly reduced human ills; now the major ills have become genetic and congenital. They can be reduced by medical controls. We ought to protect our families from the emotional and material burden of such diseased individuals, and from the misery of their simply "existing" (not *living*) in a nearby "warehouse" or public institution.

We have an example in hemophilia. If a man has a recessive gene for it, even though he himself is all right, he passes it on—not to his sons but to his daughters. They won't have the disease (it is sex-linked) but they will pass it on to their children. By controlling his reproduction through sex selection or pre-emptive abortion, keeping only male embryos, this man would stop the scourge once and for all in his family line. That is his moral responsibility.

If the State is morally justified in repelling an unwelcome invader, why should not a woman do so when burdened or invaded by an unwelcome pregnancy? And why shouldn't the family be protected from an idiot or terribly diseased sibling? Control is human and rational; submission, the opposite of control, is subhuman. Suffering and misfortune cannot be utterly escaped, it is true, and human beings can grow tremendously in pain and disappointment. But a basic ethical principle of medicine and health care is nonetheless the minimization of human suffering, by deliberate control.

Producing our children by "sexual roulette" without preconceptive and uterine control, simply taking "pot luck" from random sexual combinations, is irresponsible—now that we can be genetically selective and know how to monitor against congenital infirmities. As we learn to direct mutations medically we should do so. Not to control when we can is immoral. This way it will be much easier to assure our children that they really are here because they were *wanted*, that they were born "on purpose."

Controlling the quality of life is not negative; it just rejects what fails to come up to a positive standard. The new biology equips us to save and improve the defective, as well as to maintain a sensible standard. For example, it was once prohibitively expensive to correct dwarfism when HGH (human growth hormone) had to be extracted from human pituitaries at autopsy, but biochemistry has synthesized HGH and one day soon it will be available economically. (Such achievements are undesirable only if we allow the dwarfs we treat to pass their genetic defect along to innocent progeny.)

We began our human history by learning to control the physical environment (and still make serious mistakes). We have made some progress in controlling our social life, and we are learning to control our behavior. It is time, then, that we accepted control of our heredity.

Costs and Benefits

The essence of tragedy is the conflict of one good with another. The conflict of good with evil is only melodrama. We often have to calculate the relative desirability of things. We pay for what we get, always. Choosing high quality fetuses and rejecting low quality ones is not tragedy; sad, but not agonizing.

A heavier trial of the spirit and a real test of responsible judgment, if we want to exert serious control, would be a problem like deciding whether to induce abortion when only one of a pair of nonidentical twins has an untreatable metabolic disorder. It would mean losing a good baby to prevent a bad one. But even here compassionate control should not hesitate: the good one is still only potential, and pregnancy could—at least ordinarily—be restarted. It is far more callous not to prevent the fate of a foreseeably diseased baby than it is disappointing to postpone a good one for a matter of only months.

To be responsible, to take control and reject low quality life, only seems cruel or callous to the morally superficial. Actually, it is practical compassion. Robert Louis Stevenson was shocked at first when he found the Polynesians practicing "infanticide." Their ignorance of contraception and obstetrics meant they had to resort to "abortion at birth" when a newborn turned out to be defective, or when the small atolls they lived on simply could not yield food and shelter for any more people. It was loving concern for *actual* children in their radically finite world which led them to abortion and population control; a matter of costs and benefits.

Stevenson said, somewhat bemused, that never had he seen people anywhere who loved their children as much as those coral reef dwellers did. Of course. The world's finiteness is harder to hide on a Pacific coral reef.

Not to control, and not to weigh one thing against another, would be subhuman. A mature ethics is social, not egocentric. Call it what you will—mathematical morality, ethical arithmetic, moral calculus—we are obliged in conscience to think of benefits relative to costs.

Trying to be responsible we have to calculate. We issue drivers' licenses, for example, even though the cars of some will become lethal weapons; it is the price we pay for motor transport. If we could tell which applicants for a license will be killers we would not license them. It used to be that we had no way of knowing which couples were carrying a common gene defect or which pregnancies were positive for it. But now we *can* know; we have lost that excuse for taking genetic risks. To go right ahead with coital reproduction in many couples' cases is like walking down a line of children blindfolded and deliberately maiming every fourth child. It is cruel and insane to deprive normal but disadvantaged children of the care we could give them with the $1,500,000,000 we spend in public costs for preventable retardates.

Ethics is not loftily independent of economics and utilitarian or distributive justice. Economics deals with preferences among competing choices, and utility aims at spreading expectable benefits. What we need morally is a telescope, not just a microscope.

Cryogenics

There is no ethical reason, at least in principle, not to keep vital human tissue "on ice." The use of cryogens (low temperature agents) is practical or applied physics, bioengineering, put to work in the freeze-storage of sperm—and eventually of ova and even embryos. (Its workability and value for *whole* human bodies is still very speculative.)

In particular cases cryogenics is easily justifiable for

treatment reasons. Because a married man has oli-
gospermia his sperm might be collected over a period
of time, to aggregate it for fertilization. In another
situation he might bank it for a future marriage because he faces a sterilizing operation, either for therapeutic reasons or as a method of voluntary birth
control. A wife may be ill and temporarily unable to
"carry" a conceptus at just the time when the husband
learns of the need for the operation. Stored semen
could be used for several inseminations at the ovulation
period, thus increasing the chances of a hoped-for
conception. As laboratory fertilization develops, the
relevance and utility of banked germ plasm is obvious.
It will also be a helpful adjunct to cloning.

Cryogenics could be simple fertility insurance for
those who are going to war or other dangerous enter-
prises, and for those who work near nuclear power
piles or who risk irradiation on a nuclear submarine or
commercial freighter. Telegenesis (baby making from
germ cells stored in order to conceive when a partner
is far away) is one class of its uses, and paleogenesis
(for those separated by time—even by death) is another. Sterilization, the most reliable method of contraception, need no longer entail inevitable childlessness, now that we have cryogenics; a combination of
both sterilization *and* fertility is possible now.

The voluntary choice of germ plasm, that is, of one's
children's biological quality, is a great boon. It but-
tresses quality control and, like genetic mutations,
helps heredity to be rational and responsible.[4] Storage
banks will carry descriptions, even the names of the
donors of sperm, eggs, and embryos. "Celebrity Seed
for Sale," one wag has suggested for the display
signs.[5] Since it is done through these organized banks,
involving physicians and nurses, conceptions from
storage will have to give up the secrecy and anonymity

of some of the past practice of artificial insemination. Too many people will have to be "in the know." Candor is better than deception.

Sensible regulatory laws and policies will need to be worked out, to set guidelines. Should corporations as well as individuals be allowed to get germs or embryos, to artificially produce children? Could a "fictitious person" be a proper parent? Should we allow a business or any other such entity to produce its own labor force, bypassing the "labor market"? Should we encourage monetary payment to donors of bank-distributed germ cells and embryos—it is done already in some clinical procedures? Would clients ever have any right to return, reject, or pass on to others what they receive from a bank? Must they only be the reproducers? These are some of the legal and prudential questions at stake; there are others, of course—but apart from contingent questions like these there is no ethical objection to cryogenics as such.

Donating—Giving—Sharing

"It is more blessed to give than to receive," said Jesus. This is a moral sentiment that certainly needs no defense. Artificial insemination, egg transfers, gonad transplants, substitute gestation, and the like, now make it possible to put our generosities very close to home—in one's very own person. How "blessed" it was, to get down to cases, of the forty-five-year-old mother in Greece in 1973 who gave up her vagina for transplant to her twenty-one-year-old daughter, a victim of vaginal atresia, whose marriage was saved by the graft.[6]

Narcissism, egoism, and selfishness have heretofore had at least one last refuge that could never be threatened—one's own private and exclusive reproductivity. Every one of us either had it all to himself or herself, or lacked it altogether and were without hope. Now we can and will be asked to share our reproductivity with others, if they should lack fertility or have the wrong kind. The old alibis for the old selfishness are shot down, gone for good.

Unless there are foreseeably undesirable consequences in a particular case, we *ought* upon occasion to be donors of germ cells, gonads, or, in the case of women, of hostess gestation. It would be selfish to be sterilized by a simple tubal section, for example, if excision and transplant of the gonads could help a sterile neighbor to have a child. If we have a chance to donate one of our paired organs, should we not? Generosity and human community now have a richer range and depth. Whether or not we ourselves choose to be reproducers—by whatever method—we can and should help our friends and neighbors if they need to share our reproductivity. This is the meaning of the Roman nuns' donation of urine to facilitate the preparation of FSH. If we have acceptable help to give— no matter if we are married or not, celibate or not, parents or not—our obligation is to give it.

Ectogenesis: Outside the Womb

Nonvivaporous birds and animals lay their eggs and tend them until they hatch (are born)—it is all done outside the parents' bodies. Humans can do this too, for humane reasons and for quality's sake. If a wetnurse can supply another woman's child with her milk, and if we can give our blood to others, then how could there be any moral barrier to donating even more basic gifts, such as germ cells and placental sustenance, in hostess gestation?

No doubt trivial reasons will be given for extrauterine gestation sometimes ("I'd like to keep my figure"), but there will be more substantial reasons, too. Yet surely it is not necessary to have a solemn or highly exigent reason. Mothers are entitled to decide against using their own wombs even though the great majority will probably always opt for gestation as an important part of becoming a mother. Besides physical conditions that call for ectogenesis—serious genetic disorders, incorrigible infertility, hysterectomy, chronic heart disease, blocked tubes—there are personal vocational reasons as well.

Transcending these difficulties does *not* make mothers "obsolescent," as some have suggested. In Huxley's *Brave New World* normal birth with its physiological pain was never openly mentioned. Is such pain desirable for any real reason, other than a masochistic urge and "because the Bible says it's so" (Genesis 3:16)? As the Peking newspaper *Jenmin Jin Pao* put it, "Nine months of pregnancy is no light or easy burden and such diseases as poisoning due to pregnancy are detrimental to health. If children can be had without being borne, working mothers need not be affected by childbirth. This is happy news for women."[7]

Plastic, glass, or steel wombs, as an alternative for substitute (hostess) human carrywomen, will soon become "operational"—once we compound artificial placentas. Biochemistry has yet to work through the problem of the placenta, to figure out the chemistry of "nature." It is easy, alas, to underestimate the problem. J. B. S. Haldane wildly predicted in his little book *Daedalus* (1923) that by 1968 France would have sixty thousand babies by ectogenesis.

The glass womb is after all nothing more than an extension of the "extracorporeal membrane oxygenator," the incubator which already feeds "preemies" and babies with hyaline membrane disease. An artificial placenta, like a heart-lung machine, is a substitute for a natural function; it provides amniotic fluid chemically. Glass wombs are a radical version of early Caesarean sections. With artificial placentas we could save a fetus which might otherwise have to be lost in a medical abortion; both the patient *and the baby* could be saved. If we can save people with kidney failure by putting them on machines (artificial kidneys), and people with heart disease by putting machines in them (artificial hearts), why not do the same for *potential* people? When cloning becomes fully operational for humans, ectogenesis would in some situations eliminate the reimplantation stage, to advantage.

As in cryogenics, there will be regulatory questions. Is the genetic mother of a baby gestated by a hostess the "real" mother in the eyes of the law, or is the gestator? For example, should hostess gestators be married or single; would their husbands have veto powers; what, if any, would be the legal rights of the surrogates? These are all matters of social policy, and yet to be carefully thought through.

Egg Transfers

Egg grafts or artificial enovulations from a donor would be perfectly ethical if a person is, for example, without ovaries or has a hopeless infection of her tubes, or if she fears to pass on a genetic disease. A transfer is psychologically happier than AID because the husband is the genetic father and the wife can at least "carry" her own baby if she wants. But the *method* is more complicated—for example, getting her and the donor's ovulation periods together. Furthermore, the donor's time and discomfort is markedly greater than in AID.

Present feasibilities favor *in vitro* fertilization before the implantation of borrowed ova, rather than *in vivo* fertilization in coitus. In February 1970 a couple went to Edwards and Steptoe in England for an *in vitro* fertilization and implantation, even though the procedure is still tentative. The patient's tubes were blocked and her own ova, not a donor's, were to be used. Somehow it was aired on the BBC and a great "debate" arose. Reactionaries and sensationalists used put-down language, such as "Guinea Pig Mother of Test Tube Baby." It was said that they should be refused the investigative treatment they wanted because it is unethical, irreligious, and an unnatural medical service.

A leading Methodist ethicist countered that it was morally all right if no harm was done to the zygote. That condition is of course impossible to meet. The clinicians can be confident only that whenever their procedure results in a defective conceptus they should do what nature does when the *natural* process produces a defective conceptus—abort it, and try again.

To the warning that this artificial reproduction is playing God and is irreverent, an Anglican bishop quite wisely said, "The church would not want any restrictions imposed upon research into the beginning of life and it is certain that the outcome will never undermine belief in God as the creator."

Family and Marriage

Women who had never copulated will have children, and women who have often copulated will never have children. Babies without sex, sex without babies. Some children will have only one parent—a parent who may be either a man or a woman. Bachelor mothers and fathers will become more common. Single parents are already having children. Marriages will be contracted less often than in the past. Families, at least nuclear families, are sure to be smaller in size or frequency.

How far do we want to depart from the conventional and familiar marriage syndrome—monogamous, permanent, exclusive, heterosexual? With the separation of love making from baby making, plus the reduction of progeny numbers and the escape of women from the baby-machine role, the family is losing some of its pragmatic importance. Historically marriage and the family, which "began as a physical union and then became a legal one—to give men property rights in women and their offspring—has now reached the threshold of a moral union: a free one, elective to start, and elective to stop."[8]

The family functions primarily for the sake of the children, and rightly so; they create it. A childless couple is a "hominid pair bond," not a family. Under the influences of the new biology and social change the family's shape will change too. (Recall, for example, Alvin Toffler's futuristic option of pro-parents or professional child-rearers, in relation to bio-parents or those who generate the child.[9])

Nostalgic critics see these emerging patterns as a moral decline, a weakening of the family. One such critic even thinks we are disastrously "creating a new conception of what it means to be human." But the essence of the family—adults giving loving personal care to children—will be basically unchanged by new modes of reproduction. Children will still have ancestors, parents, siblings. The new biology only enlarges the family and deepens what it means to be human. We cannot repeat it too often; new and refined modes

of reproduction are still thoroughly biological and natural—and because they are highly rational and purposive, not just sexual roulette or marital lottery,
they are more fully human, as well as more humane.

With artificial insemination and egg transfer children are truly chosen, definitely wanted. No happen-
stance about it. By comparison, "normal" parents are
far more apt to be casual or flighty. It has been found,
for example, that there is only one divorce in 800 AID
couples compared to one divorce in every four couples
of the general population.[10]

What an extraordinary *volte face* it is for Christians
to have turned and twisted along a line from St. Paul's
legalistic claim that the only reason for marriage is
that it legitimates sex ("better to marry than to
burn") to St. Augustine's insistence that the only excuse for sex is that babies are made by means of it
(a very antisexual posture indeed) to the present-day
reactionary view of typical objectors to noncoital
asexual reproduction—the reverse opinion, now, that
the only justification for babies is that they come from
sex.

Genetic Engineering

Of all phases of the new molecular biology and reproductive medicine, what we call "genetic engineering" is furthest from being "operational" or in
practical use. Genetic intervention in humans to eliminate inborn physical and mental defects is not here
yet. But it looms ahead. Since Crick and Watson de-
ciphered DNA's three dimension double-helix base-
pair structure more than twenty years ago we have
already seen the nucleic acid code broken, then an
active viral gene synthesized, and at the practical level

the green revolution's genetic production of super-cereals and miracle rice in the "hungry Third World."

Morally, genetic engineering is good when it serves human needs, both health and happiness. If genetic manipulation were not possible in agriculture and plant physiology we would be back where Stalin and Lysenko stalled Soviet biology. If we were unable to do it in animal husbandry we would have to say good-bye to the rational reproduction of meat, work and hide animals, livestock improvement, and so on. These farming and herding techniques are for human benefit, and there is no ethical cut-off point at which to clamp an arbitrary stop on the use of genetic controls for the health and quality of human beings themselves.

Two different uses are up for approval: therapeutic or medical treatment, and the *design* of genotypes preconceptively. While some people object to all genetic intervention, others only object to genetically designing human beings—not to repairing genetic faults *after* they are conceived or born. In short, they justify it for treatment but not for prevention.

This is somewhat more humane than the blanket condemnations but hardly any more rational. It is absurd to be willing to cure human ills or lacks but unwilling to avoid or supply them before they afflict us. Such a strange posture is ethical nonsense. For example, in the relatively benign area of cosmetic surgery for disfiguring physical traits, who would prefer to have it done over and over again from generation to generation when it could be obviated once and for all by genetic intervention?

Still others would condemn any use of genetic controls to produce a "strain" of men with long arms to fit them to be orchard workers, or to produce a family of people with oversize lungs for sponge fishing or pearl diving.

Ethical questions are raised about using genetic control to choose the phenotypes of *future* individuals.* But this is after all only another version of the ethical questions we are already facing when we reproduce with known traits. We have always had to weigh the cost of our choices and purposes against our needs, and we always will. The only change would be for the good, because we would have more control with which to do what we think is right.

A sensible policy is to breed animals for special purposes instead of humans, where possible, if the specialization delimits human capacities. Dolphins, fish, pigeons, primates are even now being used to do dull or dangerous work for us. We could even design species from scratch. There is no need to drag humans down genetically to do special or menial jobs; we can bring animals *up*, to do them. As Sir George Thompson sees it, "Very large modifications in the wild species can no doubt be made."[12] For example, animal brains can be markedly improved by doses of the twenty-first human chromosome. And rather than providing people with low I.Q.s to do dull work we might take Shaw's advice (*The Intelligent Woman's Guide to Socialism*) and pay normal people extra-high wages to do what most of us don't want to do.

Human Beings, Being Human

Human beings, in order to qualify as human, have to be something more than just biologically classifiable

---

* Gerald Feinberg has put it neatly. Much as we dislike making plans which restrict the freedom of future generations, we cannot escape doing so. "An inescapable result of the one-way flow of time is that we are born into a world we never made." He adds, "I do not think that any new moral principle is established" when we exercise our honest judgment about what is best for our descendants.[11]

as organisms of the species *homo sapiens*. They have to have individual or separate existence ("viability") and they have to be actually "sapient"—that is, possessed of a functioning cerebral cortex—some minimal level of intelligence.

Therefore an individual of the species who is not yet human, a fetus, and one who has ceased to be, a "brain dead" patient, is without the status of being human or of human being. The sadness of abortion is that it means letting a potential go—but it is only a potential, not a reality; the sadness of "pulling the plug" on an irreversibly comatose patient is that it means accepting the bitter fact of a loss—acknowledging that a human being is now no more. But the point is that abortion and "brain death" terminations are *biocide*, not homicide. All talk of "killing a human being" in such cases is therefore ethically off the track.

Incidentally, the nearest thing to a specifiable "moment" for *becoming* human is when a fetus is respirated after birth—that reflexive and explosive gulp of air starting the lungs to work. This is what Plato contended. Only on his terms can it make sense to speak of the "moment" of becoming human. The "moment" of death, of *ceasing* to be human, is quite commonly unspecifiable. In any case, being human is two things essentially—intelligence and "going it alone" as an individual on one's own lungs.

Hybrids

But hold on. What if an ape had the intelligence and sensibilities of a human, and a human had only the capabilities of an ape? Which would be the human being? The answer is plain; the ape would be the human being.

This is no mere play on words. All mammals, man among them, are remarkably close biologically. Modern biology can devise "chimeras" or combinations of humans and animals, and also "cyborgs" or combinations of humans and machines. Gerald Leach warns us against the Minotaur, a mythical creature half man and half bull who was hidden away because it was too horrible to look upon.[13] The basic fact is that the body cells of all species will cross-fuse, and the germ cells of many—though not all—will unite sexually.

If a prosthetic device, perhaps an intricate mechanical hand or leg, supplies a person with 50 per cent or more of the function lost in an amputation, that is morally good. An artificial kidney or hemodialysis machine is morally good. This applies equally to heart pacemakers, dacron arteries, metal bones, ceramic hipjoints. All such technical contrivances are cyborgs or man-machine "hybrids."

Man-animal combinations are in the same ethical class. If a cow's kidney is "grown" into a patient's thigh to help cleanse his blood, after his own kidney function is gone, that is morally good. If an animal's organ or tissue is used to replace something lost by a human (an interspecific transplant) that is good. These are examples of man-animal combinations for medical purposes. And the day may come when replacement medicine will be keeping herds of animals on hand, to supply physicians with what they need. It would mean more "live" rather than transshipped cadaver transplants, and it would relieve human beings of the risks or inconveniences of the donor role.

But what of hybridization for nonmedical reasons? Chimeras or parahumans might legitimately be fashioned to do dangerous or demeaning jobs. As it is

now, low grade work is shoved off on moronic and retarded individuals, the victims of uncontrolled reproduction. Should we not "program" such workers
thoughtfully instead of accidentally, by means of hybridization? Cell fusion and putting human cell nuclei
into animal tissue is possible (such hybrid tissue exists
already as a matter of fact).

Hybrids could also be designed by sexual reproduction, as between apes and humans. If interspecific
coitus is too distasteful, then laboratory fertilization
and implant could do it. If women are unwilling to
gestate hybrids animal females could. Actually, the
artificial womb would bypass all such repugnances. In
some cases even the sterility of hybrids might be overcome. (Euphenic changes, such as cell fusion tissues
would be, are not transmissible genetically.)

Contrived in order to protect human beings from
danger, a social reason, or from disease, a medical reason, chimeras and cyborgs would be morally justified.
What counts is human need and well-being.

Incest

The prohibition of incest among humans is a fictive
(in the sense of a nonbiological) rule. It exists for socially pragmatic reasons. On the whole it has been a
good rule. It has enforced a healthy "exogamy" or marriage outside the group or family, with a consequent
variation of human genotypes—resulting from the input of different strains. Also it has the effect of distributing wealth and spreading power.

Other animals have no aversion to incest, and
breeders often reinforce their livestock's natural in-
cestuousness for quality purposes. The so-called "in-

stinct" against incest is a matter of cultural conditioning, not a biologically based aversion. Religious claims that it is against "nature" or the "laws of nature" are groundless. Brother-sister reproduction goes on on a wide scale all of the time, occasionally even among human beings. Exogamy or outbreeding is a sound policy for distributing bad genes and avoiding the locked-in concentration of faults which has ruined famous families such as the Jukes and Kallikaks and some royal family lines. In the same way endogamy or inbreeding is a sound policy for holding good genes together and preserving superior genotypes—provided, of course, that the "strain" does not include too many subfaults which might aggregate and subvert the good qualities.

Warnings that artificial insemination might end up in incest have no biological force. As a matter of fact, the statistics are that there would be only one occurrence in fifty to a hundred years, at the rate of two thousand AIDs performed per year, if each donor contributed only five times. And clonants, having the same sex as the parent cell, could not possibly engage in incest with a fellow clonant—unless it was homosexual incest.

We have here a case of conduct in which there is nothing inherently or absolutely wrong, yet the greatest good of the greatest number might best be served by disapproving it. Having said as much, however, we may then hold that in particular cases it could be right to practice incest. It would depend on the situation, presumably an odd and highly unusual situation. The only argument against meeting human needs in such cases, other than the *a priori* "law of nature," would have to be the slippery slope or wedge argument—that *any* exceptions at all to the rule would lead to abandoning its wisdom as a general policy. This would be hard to make stick, just as it is in surgery in spite of "do the patient no harm" or executive clemency in spite of "criminals should pay for their crimes."

Trying to imagine situations where incest would be desirable, even if tolerable, is exceedingly difficult. But there is an important difference ethically; incest is tolerable because it is not in and of itself an evil, even though it would only rarely be possible to show that it is positively desirable. The main point is: Instead of twisting biology to fit an ethical system, let's build our ethics to fit biology and human well-being.

Love Making

Love as an interpersonal sentiment is of course wider and deeper than sexual intercourse, just as "sexuality" is. But in the restricted sense of intercourse "love making," like other human acts, is not inherently either right or wrong. Our moral judgments on sex acts are determined by many extrinsic and contextual variables—such factors as the intentions and attitudes of the parties, their marital status or lack of it, their health, their age and competence, and so on.

If we keep two crucial realities in mind—the separation biologically of love making from baby making, and the critical need socially and ecologically to arrest or even reverse population growth—we will see that our moral scheme must have a place for sex freedom and variety. Love making has a two-dimensional nature, "procreation and recreation." On its procreative side, sex should be well controlled, a discipline of careful calculation, whether it is carried out naturally or artificially. On its recreative side, spontaneity and personal feeling should reign.

Women are not baby machines, men are not baby machine operators, and homes are not human manufacturing plants. Women are persons first of all, not wives or spinsters. Fathers-in-law no longer require a bride price from husbands, nor do they lose it if the bride is not a virgin. Virginity (a condition) as distinguished from chastity (a virtue) is not so much valued any more. Spouses (especially wives) are no longer private property; husbands no longer bury two or three wives in a lifetime. Legalistic language like "the marital debt" does not fit authentic love making.

Terms which tie love making so closely to marriage —we speak of premarital, comarital and extramarital sex—are archaic. They reflect an outmoded inflexibility of sexual role, too stereotyped to fit our deepening sense of personal freedom and responsibility. (Francoeur lists as many as twenty telltale variants in patterned sexual behavior.[14]) More and more people remain single, and extramarital sex or "adultery" increases, as among the retired elderly who often have very practical reasons for not marrying—and aren't really expected to. The blackmailing business, to put it another way, is in decline.

Heterosexual, monogamous, permanent, and sexually exclusive marriage still remains an ideal and a reality for many and possibly even for most people. At the same time, divorce figures indicate a general acceptance of serial polygamy—as being more humane than a relentless maintenance of one-shot monogamy, regardless of the unhappiness of the partners.

Reproduction will be moving away to some extent from sexual intercourse and marriage is losing its old simplistic foundation. We must either find new moral guidelines for old values—or change our values.

Parenthood

Mothers and fathers are of several different kinds now. Take mothers: Some are genetic (they provide the egg), some are natal (they carry the fetus), some are social (they rear or "bring up" the child). All of them can play a part in a child's creation—yet no one of them needs to fill more than one of these roles. All of them, or any combination, would be ethical as far as the functions themselves are concerned.

Parental (and kin) relationships need to be reconceptualized. They cannot any more be based on blood or wombs or even genes. Parenthood will have to be understood nonbiologically or, to be specific, *morally*. Its own achievements have forced biology out of court in validating parental relations. The mere fact of conceiving a child or donating the elements of its conception or gestating it does not establish anybody as a father or a mother. Parental love has by this time become truly interpersonal; no longer can it be merely germinal, somatic, or physiological—and certainly not merely genital. An authentic parental bond is established morally, by care and concern, not by some simple physicalist doctrine.

Uterine and ovarian transplants, like egg and embryo transfers, further extend the legalistic questions about paternal rights raised nearly fifty years ago when AID was started. Maternity now is in question too, as paternity used to be. The old rule that only paternity is not self-evident (*"Mater semper certa est, pater est quem nuptiae demonstrat"*) is overthrown by reproductive medicine.

Morally, donors of seed or ova ought to have no

claims of any kind on recipient or child, nor recipient or child on a donor, nor recipient or child on the spouses of either a donor or a recipient. What counts morally is the commitment of the participants, not what they contribute. All of this complexity forces us to embrace a moral rather than physical definition of parenthood.

Research and Ignorance

The geneticist Joshua Lederberg said in his paper at the Nobel symposium in Stockholm in September 1969 ("Orthobiosis, the Perfection of Man"), "The suppression of knowledge appears to me unthinkable, not only on ideological but on merely logical grounds. How can the ignorant know what they should not know?"[15]

Dr. Lederberg's remark is aimed at those who want to suppress research because they are afraid of "dangerous" knowledge, especially in the field of human reproduction. It may be conceded that we ought not to embark on irreversible innovations if we are sure we know them to be both irreversible and imprudently dangerous—such things (presumably) as immortality pills, untraceable poisons, or a hydrogen bomb that could be made in private bedrooms. The new biology, however, is not of that caliber or character.

"The answer to dangerous knowledge," as Van Rensselaer Potter has noted, "continues to be more knowledge."[16] Deliberately to choose ignorance is unethical, immoral. It is comforting, therefore, to recall that the risks of damage to *in vitro* conceptions and implanted embryos is no greater than the errors in natural or *in vivo* pregnancies; neither is risk free.

A related moral issue is raised around the research

use of live fetuses obtained from either medically prescribed or personally elected abortions. "Right to life"
or "pro-life" agitators in 1973 actually intimidated the
U. S. National Institutes of Health into (at least temporarily) suspending their approval of many programs
of research into the causes of genetic and fetal disorders. On the other hand, a conference of Britain's
leading obstetricians, chaired by Sir John Peel, settled in
1972 on a fairly sensible policy, ethically regarded—
although at some points it shows more compromise
than logic.[17] An inviable fetus (less than five months)
and fetal material at any stage (placenta, fluids,
membranes) may be used. Nothing is said in their
policy statement, incidentally, about any "rights" of
the fetus. A good deal is quite properly said about the
patient's rights of consent or objection.

It is contended that an abortee's permission should
be given before any use is made of her fetus or fetal
material and this would seem ordinarily to be the
right principle. But surely this limiting principle could
be disregarded in some situations—for example, when
a woman stubbornly refuses consent even though her
fetus holds a promising clue to an epidemic or, equally
hypothetical, if it were discovered that the abortus
contains an agent that will cure or control cancer. The
antiabortionists, of course, object to postabortional
fetal research even if the patient's permission is given,
and no matter what the excuse.

Rights and Regulation

All alleged human rights cease to be right, become
unjust, when their exercise would victimize innocent
third parties and bystanders. All rights are "imperfect,"

not absolute or uncontingent. We might say this particularly of the so-called "right to privacy" as it bears on propagating at will and inordinately. The social welfare and protection of third parties has a prior claim. The "right" to reproduce, like all others, is—morally weighed—really only a privilege.

A worrisome side to the practice of control is whether it should ever be imposed or must always be voluntary. If people could be relied upon to be compassionate we would have no reason to even consider mandatory controls. But there are too many who do not control their lives out of moral concern; they are self-centered about what they do or neglect to do, even though they may be "cagey" about it. Large families and a pious disregard of genetic counseling, like refusing to undergo vaccinations until it is made a matter of police enforcement, show how the common welfare often has to be safeguarded by compulsory control or what Garrett Hardin calls "mutual coercion mutually agreed upon."[18]

Coercion is a dirty word to liberals, but all social controls—e.g., the government's tax powers—are really what the majority agree upon, however reluctantly, out of enlightened self-interest and a *quid pro quo* willingness to give up something to get something better. It might be protection from overpopulation, for instance. Ideally it is better to do the moral thing freely, but sometimes it is more compassionate to force it to be done than to sacrifice the well-being of the many to the egocentric "rights" of the few. This obviously is the ethics of a sane society. Compulsory controls on reproduction would not, of course, fit present interpretations of due process in the fifth and fourteenth amendments to the Constitution.[19] Here, as in so many other ways, the law lags behind the ethics of modern medicine and public health knowledge.

Screening

A good illustration of the tension between rights and regulation takes shape in trying to control hereditary disease. Each of us carries from five to ten genetic faults. If they match up in sexual roulette, tragedy results. How can we avoid or curtail the danger? Denmark prohibits marriages of certain couples unless they are sterilized. But if this method of control and prevention is used, or any other, how do we find out *who* are the ones who should not marry or, if they do, should not have babies by the natural or coital mode? Screening by one means or another is the obvious way to fulfill our obligation to potential children, as well as to the community which has to suffer when defectives are born.

The law in most countries is far behind our emerging medical information. People are not required to make their bad genes known to their mates nor are physicians required to reveal the facts. A man with polycystic kidney disease is not required to let it be known—even though it is highly immoral (unjust) to keep knowledge of such a hereditary disaster (renal failure in middle age) from his children and those they marry. Medical genetics will continue to isolate more and more such diseases, so that as our ability to prevent disease and tragedy increases so does the moral guilt of secrecy, indifference to the consequences for others, and fatalistic inaction.

Conquering infectious diseases reduces the cause of the trouble, but to conquer genetic diseases *increases* the cause or source of the trouble. This dysgenic effect is the first big-scale moral dilemma for medicine—truly a dilemma. Infections come from the environment around us but genetic faults come from within us, and therefore any line of genetic sufferers allowed to propagate will spread their disease through more and more carriers. As we cut down on the infectious diseases we are threatened with a relative rise in deaths and debility due to genetic disorders. We are now approaching a situation in which genetic causes account for as many *or more* deaths than "disease" in the popular sense.

Our moral obligation to undergo voluntary screening, if it is indicated, is too obvious to underline. The squeeze here, ethically, is that the social good often requires *mass* screening. When it is voluntary it is "nicer," as we see in the popular acceptance of tests for cervical cancer. But let it be compulsory if need be, for the common good—Hardin's "mutual coercion mutually agreed upon." Francis Crick has said that "if we can get across to people the idea that their children are not entirely their own business and that it is not a private matter, it would be an enormous step forward."[20] The biophysicist Leroy Augenstein estimated in 1972 that a total of 6 per cent of births or one out of seventeen, are defective. Of these, he said, forty thousand to fifty thousand children every year "are so defective that they don't know that they are human beings."[21] His figures are more impressive than his formulation, however; if an individual cannot "know" he is a human being he is not a human being.

Parents of adopted children and donors of AID are much more carefully screened and selected than "natural" parents—which is logically ridiculous even though we can understand how it came about. A socially conscientious system would be a national registry; blood and skin tests done routinely at birth and fed into a computer-gene scanner would pick up all anomalies, and they would be printed out on data cards and filed; then when marriage licenses are applied for, the cards would be read in comparison machines to find incompatibilities and homozygous conditions.

The objection is, predictably, that it would "violate" a "right"—the right to privacy. It is even said, in a brazen attack on reason itself, that we have a "right to *not* know." Which is more important, the alleged "privacy" or the good of the couple as well as of their progeny and society? (The couple could unite anyway, of course, but on the condition Denmark makes—that sterilization is done for one or both of them. And they could even still have children by medical and donor assistance, bypassing their own faulty fertility.)

Screening is no more an invasion of privacy than "contact tracing" in the treatment of venereal disease, or income tax and public health records, or compulsory fluoridation of the water, or the age-old codes of consanguinity (which were only based on nonsense). A good education for those who balk would be a week's stay in the wards of a state institution for the "retarded"—a term used to cover a host of terrible distortions of humanity. Just let them *see* the nature and extent of it; that would convince them.

Sex Selection

The ethical issues raised about preselection of children's sex are mainly two: whether it is wrong to exercise that much control over our progeny, and whether it is right to throw the sex ratio out of balance. The second "issue" is based on an assumption that most people would prefer boys to girls.

By way of answering, we would say that control as such is good, not evil, and the more the better, but that it should not be used for immoral purposes. Throwing the sex ratio out of near balance might be undesirable if it denied some people their aliquot share of sexual partnership. This could be the case in a strictly monogamous culture, even though single persons and celibates (to say nothing of group-marriage members) could have children asexually. With fewer progeny needed or wanted, and sexual intercourse freer in part because of that fact, there is now much less need for a near balance of the sexes. And in the last resort, reproduction no longer will have to depend on marital-coital-gestational reproduction.

The assumption that the male gender is better and more desirable is a bare-faced piece of male chauvinism and androcentric psychology. To suppose that fetal sex choice and freedom of abortion would mean throwing out "worthless females" is both hilarious and foolish. If men were stupid enough to do it (they aren't) the women would soon set things straight.

There is also the related issue, the assertion that embryos are human beings and that superfetation and selection is "mass murder." This strident protest is not ethically tenable. Even its metaphysical validity is dubious, to say nothing of its unethical and antimedical consequences if it were followed out logically.

Sterilization

In May 1973 the Supreme Court upheld a lower court's decision that it was unconstitutional when the Worcester (Massachusetts) City Hospital denied a patient's request for a voluntary sterilization. That settled the legal side of it.

On the ethical side sterilization is plainly a matter of personal freedom and responsibility. It is as moral a means to the end as any other form of birth control. In fact, its reliability makes it more responsible. Sterilization is not absolutely ethical, of course. Nothing is. But unless it either violates a promise or denies some real obligation to propagate (which would be rare situations indeed) it is morally right.

As a matter of fact, even after a woman has had a sterilization she could still have children. Once we worried about the irreversibility of sterilization. But now a woman can have the tubes finally closed off, yet aspirate the eggs by laparascope, fertilize them *in vitro*, and then have one egg implanted in her own womb for nurture. We could drop vasectomies and the pill, and practically eliminate any abortions except those done for therapeutic and genetic reasons.

Value, Values

Human acts and things are both like poker chips, they have whatever value or worth we—human beings —choose to assign to them. A red one is worth so much, a blue one so much, a white one so much. Put negatively, nothing has intrinsic value—things have no value apart from how human beings feel about them. As in games where chips are used, so in real affairs we agree about the relative values of what we do and what we want in terms of humanly desirable and exchangeable needs and aspirations.

For example, would we on principle "bump" a suicide from an intensive care unit (ICU) to save an auto accident victim, if it had to be one or the other? The answer, surely, is No. We cannot say that all suicides want to die, nor that all auto accident casualties want to live. It depends. Every case has to be looked at on its own merits.

How we judge or weigh our decisions in real life situations will depend on what we know or suppose we know about the alternatives. One thing we can be sure of; it is immoral in the extreme to say, as one member of the British Parliament did in the debate on the Abortion Act of 1967, "We are not here to listen to professional opinion, we are here to legislate." That posture, Don't Bother Me With the Facts, My Mind Is Made Up, is the last word in irresponsibility.

As we have seen in nearly all of our ethical problems, the pressure comes when the social interest fails to phase with the personal. The conviction throughout this book, perhaps because we believe that without survival of the species all talk about ethics is academic, is that the general welfare comes first. Look at Robert Louis Stevenson's turn-around experience. He went to Polynesia *sure* that "infanticide" is wrong. What happened to him?

Stevenson already knew "in the back of his mind" that we exist in a finite world inescapably. But he never really understood what he "knew" until he stood on a small atoll in the vast surrounding sea, trying to identify with the outlook of the inhabitants. Then he could grasp the fact that these tiny atolls are true paradigms of the finite "spaceship Earth." When too many babies were born (because the atoll dwellers did not yet know how to prevent it) they accepted the moral responsibility of "aborting at birth" *because they loved their children* and knew that there is a point of too much. He finally saw the ethical error of his simplistic prohibition of infanticide.

This may appear to be a remote example or *ultima ratio* of the relativity of values. But before we dismiss it too lightly we should hold it long enough in mind to test the ethical validity of the concepts of species survival and social conscience.

Wrongful Life

We have already reached the conclusion that sometimes it is wrong to procreate a life, but let it be nailed down again. In the law they speak of wrongful death —deaths due, for example, to criminal negligence. Now the new biology and reproductive medicine are confronting us ethically with the reality of wrongful *life*, too.

A wrongful death is one which results from a "tort" or injurious, blameworthy act for which the victim or his agents and beneficiaries should be indemnified or somehow compensated. In any case, the tort is by definition blameworthy, wrong. People who know a child will be defective, or could have known if they had cared but nonetheless allowed it to be born, are as guilty of wrongdoing as those who culpably contribute to a wrongful death.

The ethical principle, as distinct from (but not unrelated to) the legal category of wrongful death, is that there is indeed such a thing as wrongful life. Already the courts have accepted two or three suits by the victims of misconception and misgestation, or by others involved; the principle is taking form, inevitably. We are as morally responsible for what we do at the start of a life as we are for what we do at the end of it. And the test, at both the alpha and the omega on the continuum, is loving concern.

VI

SOME HOPES

Borrowing the language of Proverbs, "Where there is no vision the people perish." Perhaps a better word is prevision. Human beings are capable of foresight; it sets them apart in the animal order. They have it to profit by if they use it. That first woman, Pandora, fashioned in the beauty of Venus, and immensely curious, let many evils fly out as she lifted the lid on the box in which Prometheus had tried to lock them away. But at the bottom of the chest hope was still left. And the key ingredients of hope, which give it its triumphs, are foresight and purpose.

Things move so fast that we have to think faster. In 1970 the National Academy of Sciences invited a group to report on the amount of time it would take to put various theoretical innovations into effect. They decided, among other things, that it would be about 1995 before a human egg could be fertilized *in vitro* and then implanted in a genetic or surrogate mother. Yet in 1970 Steptoe and Edwards had the procedure already within range of clinical practicability. We simply cannot keep on slipping into the mood of those who said the automobile was "interesting" but could never replace the horse on the highway.

The synthetic chemistry and molecular biology of yesterday are curing disease today, just as the theoretical physics of yesterday provides the nuclear power of today. Only twenty years ago heredity was hidden in abstract genetic language; today it has found explicit chemical terms to work with in ameliorating human faults and constructing better bodies. These are the two main tasks of all medicine in general, of course, but genetic intervention in particular aims to repair genetic defects and to improve the genetic stock. Great expectation, great hopes, push us on. More and more, now, we are open to the implications in Konrad Lorenz's opinion that we ourselves are the "long-sought missing link" between animals and really human beings.[1] It is no longer possible to entertain a self-image as complacent as the one we used to have because we assumed we were fixed in whatever shape we were given by nature.

Isaac Asimov, the most versatile of science fictioneers, speaks with wry humor of his own profession: "Attempts to look into a crystal ball are perhaps the riskiest of occupations. Unfortunately, it is also one of the most exciting. Given the chance to prophesy, only the strongest and most level-headed individuals can resist."[2] On the other side, though, we know perfectly well that even if our glimpses into the future are blurred and opaque we still have to look as hard as we can—and that we cannot postpone it too long. There is high wisdom in the tale about the Frenchman who said to his gardener after breakfast, "Plant me a tree this afternoon." When the gardener replied, "No hurry; it won't bear fruit for at least fifteen years," the householder retorted, "Well, in that case you had better plant it this morning." To avoid stumbling into the future we have to get started soon enough.

Biological life is amazingly tough; it is we who suffer, not life, when life is ignored or supinely allowed to take its own course. Just recently a Soviet geochemist, N. Chudinov, reported from the Urals that potassium rock dissolved in distilled water had yielded up a group of Paleozoic microorganisms. This microscopic life had lain dormant 250 *million years* and yet it promptly reactivated and began to reproduce normally. Life goes on and on but men themselves may lose out, if they want the ride but won't do the driving.

A Word to the Wise

The old Romans used to say, "One augur cannot look at another augur without smiling." If this refers to their sense of humor—if it is humility and not just rascality—it should help us to keep sober about our own prophesying and futurizing. Incidentally, there are always elements of unanchored fancy, personal bias, and stubborn wish-thinking trying to seduce the prognosticator. This book's writer is only too well aware of the truth in Dennis Gabor's *bon mot*, "Any book on the future will tell more about its author than of things to come."[3] Gabor himself is a serious and competent futurist; nobody is better able than he is to detect the unavoidable personal input and yet to refuse to be paralyzed by it.

Saying this is not intended to minimize the problem. At our soberest we still need to be suspicious of easy and complacent expectations sneaking in, and we have to "second guess" every prediction, minor as well as major. Otherwise we may get what we think we want only to learn that we do not want it. Some of us find it amusing, others see it as ominous, that Aldous Huxley's fantasied pacifier to make docile slaves of people in his "brave new world"—a drug for which Huxley coined the name "soma"—is already here and in use. The *PDR* (physicians' desk reference) now actually lists a relaxant with precisely that name. There is a kind of built-in possibility of too much too soon, as well as of too little too late, and it is the former aspect which leads some temperaments to want to quit moving ahead.

Also, we must hope that technology, the ways we use our scientific knowledge, will learn or be required to be more prudent than in the past. This applies as much to medical as to industrial and agricultural technology. "We can see that while technology and science solve many human problems they also create new problems in the very process of solving the old ones. To solve these problems we must not and cannot abandon our technology; we have to use more of it. Having bitten into the fruit of the tree of knowledge, we cannot return to Eden. We have reached the end of innocence."[4]

To give one example of the balance needed, if we pursue our knowledge of replacement medicine and surgery, managing to prolong the lives of many more patients by transplants and regenerative biochemistry, but do it before we have learned how to renew or refresh the *brains* of these people, the world could soon be filled with "healthy" seniles.

The chemistry of synthetics has the potential of starting us to think in terms of human initiatives rather than of just making do with existing "biologicals" and natural resources. The Red Chinese success with insulin is such a sign of the times. Yet even here we have to be careful. Now we can save or prolong the lives of diabetics without having to rely solely on the limited supply of insulin we could extract from horses or other biological sources, but we are still faced with the question how we are to balance that off against the risk of spreading diabetes to a greatly increased number of children. Things like synthetic chemistry mean vastly greater freedom for human beings—but only if they are prudently employed by us in a wide enough systems context.

An English bishop in the late 1920s proposed a ten-year moratorium on scientific research, to let society catch up with its effects; in a way this is what Alvin Toffler seems to want in *Future Shock* when he warns us against "information overload" and "decision shock" and urges the need to control the timing and rate of change. Johannes Burger of the University of Maryland, on retirement, recommended a fifty-year moratorium on cloning, and on the same scope Lewis Mumford says he favors a "restrictive discipline."*

Though such cautions are thoughtful and called-for, it is hard nevertheless to believe that we would be safer or "better off" if we had stopped work in physics and biology in 1900. Is there any way, we wonder, other than by our subjective feelings, to establish cut-off points or to define marginal value and the point of no return? One thing seems to be coming clear—gains in the tricky business of evaluating the area of knowledge are so relative to other areas that we need generalists to cope with the complexity—with the interfaces of vital biological, technical, and social forces. Encouraging specialists to go ahead on their own, *ultra vires*, becomes at some point too hit and miss—no matter how successful they are within their own bailiwicks. Their findings have to be coordinated, and control will have to be shared.

Bertrand Russell, whose irenic intelligence kept sev-

* By cloning they do not mean the making of a "prefabricated man," incidentally. That is a careless term. Cloning is a *biological* process, and a *fabricated* man would be made of nonbiological materials—plastic, metal, leather, and electronics—and these constructs would be only pseudo-hominoids. Even a "man-machine hybrid" or cyborg is only fabricated in part—the lesser part.

eral generations on their toes, expressed a lot of reservation in the 1920s about the prospective results of the biological revolution.[5] Among other things, at that early date, he said of the separation of sex from reproduction and its possible consequences in the days ahead: "Sentiments of personal affection may still be connected with intercourse not intended to be fruitful, while impregnation will be regarded in an entirely different manner, more in the light of a surgical operation, so that it will be thought not ladylike to have it performed in the natural manner." He foresaw both quantity and quality control, but believed it would have the effect of putting an end to joy.

Given a sharp mind like Russell's, and such a sly wit, we can only deplore his failure to explain *why* he felt as he did. This question, *why* is something desirable or undesirable, the ethical question, is the most subtle and complex and fateful question we have to ask ourselves at this juncture in the world's history. Even if it turns out that we cannot reach a common mind on what is wanted, even if we disagree, nonetheless it is vital to clear up *why* we disagree. Agreeing to disagree is part of what it means to have a free society, but agreement even of this negative kind cannot be reached without being sure we understand the roots of our disagreement or without having made sure that the grounds of disagreement are not illusory.

There is probably only one adequate and insurmountable reason against trying to ask such questions or get answers: if, that is, we have no hope that any gain can be made. Dr. Catherine Roberts, a biologist, has written a book called *The Scientific Conscience* in which this negative and unhopeful attitude toward the new biology is spelled out.[6] Without hope of at least a *relative* triumph for human health and well-being the natural or logical posture is to believe that a bird in the hand is worth two in the bush. Human beings as a kind, however, are and always have been creatures of hope, the agents of hope, and the justifiers of hope. The bird that happens to be already in hand always gets old and lethargic and loses its beauty.

The Ethics Needed

What is the kind of ethics we hope for? What ethical approach do we need if our hopes are to come to anything? We have already described the essentials but now we can end with this plain-spoken acknowledgment. The moral philosopher is no longer able to be the answer giver or oracle; he acts only as a catalyst, a question poser, turning to others for the answers. Now the doers are really the ones who find the answers. Our situation biologically has passed far beyond the old precedents and beyond the packaged answers that were built upon the old folklore of life.

The Glasgow geneticist, G. Pontecorvo, put it squarely enough when he said that "present-day philosophers, systems of ethics, and religions . . . are unprepared for, and possibly unable to cope with, situations changing at an unprecedented pace."[7] When Chief Justice Warren Burger confessed that the law "lags behind the most advanced thinking in every area" and must therefore wait "until theologians, moral leaders, and events have created some common ground," he was still thinking along the old lines, but the fact is that ethicists have had to surrender their reins to the situation-changers.[8]

Professor Frank Grad of the Columbia University Law School forecasts the legal timing schedule of biological-medical issues this way: fully present—organ transplants, *in utero* medicine, and therapeutic insemination; pressing and imminent—artificial fertilization and enovulation, superfetation, cloning, and biochemical extensions of life; soon or eventually—genetic manipulation, parthenogenesis, cyborg medicine.[9] Here we have a practical sense of timing and social change, but all of it founded on a lively hope.

It is entirely practical to hope that personal quality, not just the quantity of biological life, will win general acceptance as the ideal; modern people will come to recognize with the Catholic oratorian of Naples, Mario Borelli, that the crucial moral question is not "when is the fetus human" but when is it *persona humana*?[10] A growing person-ism is behind movements such as women's liberation—there is a nearly universal repudiation of Aquinas' opinion, "Woman is misbegotten and defective."[11] Just to get down to a specific, illustrative of the general principle, wild proposals that we ought to clone human beings in order to make "spare parts" available for transplant medicine will be thrown out of court. Animals will be cloned instead—assuming that cloning is found to be the best means for that purpose (an unlikely assumption).

A dissenting opinion in the Rockefeller Commission's report on population control offers us a startling example of the kind of ethics we would *not* hope for. A teacher in a Washington, D.C., medical school insisted that (1) contraceptive help should not be available to minors, unless married or self-supporting; (2) fetuses are fully human and abortions immoral; (3) an "unborn child" has a right to life; (4) technology cannot solve human problems; (5) overpopulation is not a major problem, and (6) the size of a family is the family's "sacred trust" and up to its own discretion.[12] Here we have in a nutshell an ethos which is almost the complete antithesis of our person-centered, hope-sustained, and socially conscientious outlook.

Van Rensselaer Potter, explaining that ethical values cannot be separated from biological facts, lists a number of areas of human concern where there is need of a new and more contemporary ethics—an ethic of land use, of wildlife, population, consumption, geriatrics.[13] We can add other areas calling for new ethics: reproduction, genetics and directed mutation, transplantation, parenthood, sexual conduct, and so on. On every hand, happily, we see substantial evidence that we are awake already to the moral issues of air and water pollution (even at last the folly of sound pollution), ecology and conservation. Civilized people realize we need a rational ethics to select values and to define the "survival parameters" for both human beings and their environment.

All of these things come down essentially to the one hope which unifies all hopes—that is, the hope that we will shoulder the responsibility to control quality. The life sciences have made QOL (quality of life) the Number One moral imperative of mankind.

Even though defining and relating our values is the fundamental task of ethics, we seem to do it, when we do it at all, by only asking for a show of hands (voting). But this voting is based on "gut feeling" responses to questions about preferences. Something more carefully calculated than feeling, however, is needed to prevent babble and confusion. Take the lively arguments that run back and forth about the use of various forms of "behavior control"—psychological conditioning, drugs, brain surgery, electronic signals, and so on. The behaviorist B. F. Skinner, whose name is rightly prominent in the debate, is saying to us in effect: We ought (an ethical word) to choose (an ethical act) to be conditioned (i.e., give up what we think of as free choice) because to do so would make us happier and able more consistently to follow the virtues (an ethical term meaning behavioral value) of an enlightened society.

What Skinner proposes can be done—but *should* it be done? Must conduct be free and spontaneous, or could it be programmed and still be "ethical"? What are the virtues, and how ought they to be ranked or ordered? How do we want these questions to be settled? These are the profound questions lying beneath quality of life ethics, and they beg us for more reflective answers than they are getting. Just the same, we continue to hope that workable answers will be found; we are encouraged to hope so by signs of a new and more sophisticated awareness of the questions themselves, shown in a hundred ways.

Even with humane and compassionate motives, however, it is not by any means self-evident that we ought or that we ought not to use some of our chemical and biological controls. The case for virogenic therapy to cure cancer, if it works out, would seem to be plain and incontestable, but what about the use of a "hypno-virus" in war weaponry? It would be a bloodless form of combat, a symptomless "bullet" to shoot the enemy with, making him stupid for several days until, when he is put down and contained, we could administer the antidote—kept secret as an ace in the hole. But is there a course of ethical reasoning which could show us that it is better or worse than explosive shells and cartridges? This kind of question is no longer merely an ethical issue for science-fiction scenarios.

The new temper finds expression in an appeal by Salvador Luria, the M.I.T. biologist: "Science creates power. The uses to which this power will be put in human affairs involves choices and decisions, that is, value judgments . . . This implies a special responsibility of scientists; that of informing the public of the actual and potential application of their findings and of the possible consequences."[14]

Another hope is that in this search for quality we can keep a balance between rationality and feeling. Reason must be master or the game is lost, but without feeling and sentiment (as distinguished from sentimentality) we will lack the motive power for ethical concern. To be "truly human," to be wholesome persons, we cannot be merely "Apollonian"—all calculation and analysis and discipline and logic, nor simply "Dionysian"—just intuitive and poetic and "free!" and "gutsy." Being only visceral or only cerebral falsifies our humanness. Our true hope ethically lies in the synthesis of the two.

New ways of looking at our needs, which means our values, will show up in new ways of doing things. For instance, knowing what we do about the fertility of a single bull in relation to a herd's growth, and the need to provide more and better beef and dairy products for human beings, we will not continue much longer to keep a million bulls around eating food that a million cows and calves might have.

The reverse of this bovine *machismo* will be the standard for human males; inflating men's egos by their siring a lot of offspring will be treated as a cause for shame, not applause. Bulls will be few and fertile, but men will be many and irreproductive. On the same basis, genetic controls will inevitably bring pests and dangerous insects into a pro-human order by engineering sterility among them to stop their spread sexually (a strategy already in wide use) or by gene deletions to eliminate their pestiferous traits. This is a quality ethics at work. Cattle and insects ought to be bent to human needs; their numbers and nature ought to be subordinated to human desires—within, of course, a rational ecological balance.

Control of life for the common good will, hopefully, change our way of looking at things. We will soon see how absurd it is that we have to be issued driver's licenses to operate an automobile while we are free to go on producing children of any old kind we want or happen to conceive, without let or hindrance. And therefore among QOL policies to come we will surely have such rational controls as genetic registries, RAPIDs (an acronym for Register for Ascertaining and Preventing Inherited Disease). It is a matter of sanity—just plain sanity—to use our genetic knowledge to benefit all of the people, all of the time. This is where we are going, and where we ought to go.

Conclusion

Back in 1965 the president of the American Chemical Society asserted that since the synthesis of life itself is now within reach we should make it a national goal, similar to the manned moonshot program. Synthesis would involve the whole range of genetics and human reproduction. We have crossed a great divide; we know now that the old maxim *omne animal ex ovo* is not true, as a matter of fact. Biogenesis is no longer the whole story; life can come now from other than living sources.

There are, of course, other needs and vistas besides the biological, but deciding now to put man himself at the center of inquiry, as much and even more than his tools, makes very good sense.

With understandably mixed feelings Jean Rostand has explained, from his great eminence as a biologist, that he expects (hopes?) the artificial creation of life will come fairly soon. He calls it "causing life to be born, for the second time, of something other than itself."[15] The first genesis was a spontaneous explosion of gases; this time it will be man's achievement.

The future is not to be sought in the stars but in us, in human beings—because that is where our needs lie. There are no "acts of God" any more. Man holds himself to blame or praise for whatever happens, except so-called natural catastrophes beyond human control. It is not a world run from outside by God's will, in any case. We don't pray for rain, we irrigate and seed clouds; we don't pray for cures, we rely on medicine and the scientists who keep looking for cures until they find them. The Bible's view of the world as a shuttlecock between good and evil "powers" is meaningless, even when we admit that such language is only "mythological."

The death of the old God who was once thought to manipulate our fortunes does not, however, make things easier ethically. We ought not to underrate the heavy burden of a humanist or secular worldview. It was *easier* in the old days to attribute at least some of what happened to God's will—we could say with a moral shrug that we weren't responsible. Now we have to shoulder it all. The moral tab is ours and we have to pick it up. The excuses of ignorance and helplessness are growing thin. This is the direction of the biological revolution—that we turn more and more from creatures to creators.

We may not be as well equipped for this role as we might like to be. Human beings certainly have nothing of the omniscience people used to think God enjoyed, but even on a more humble and pragmatic level we fall short of the amount of brain capacity we could have—and may yet want to get for ourselves. The human brain at first increased rapidly but then it stopped at the Neanderthal man's size, 100,000 years ago. Why? Because the cervical or birth canal is too small to allow passage to a cranium bigger than 1,500 millimeters, less than a liquid quart. With Caesarean deliveries we could, of course, manage birth for bigger brains. But surely this is unnecessary, if indeed bigger brains were sometime to be needed, now that we can plan on the use of glass wombs—a simpler and easier delivery than human parturition can be at its best, no matter what the size or shape of the fetus.

"No one really questions, I think," said Bentley Glass, "that even now we may be like little boys on the shores of a vast ocean, tossing pebbles into the waves. What remains to be learned may dwarf imagination."[16] It is this kind of solemn intellectual humility, combined with moral courage, which, as we have seen, frightens some of us and motivates others.

Above all, we must hope that our new powers of control will not be trapped in some grandiose doctrinal or doctrinaire scheme of taking the biosphere over completely, or of serving some goal of universal salvation. Religious, Marxist, elitist—whatever the ideology—a utopianism wrapped up in a prejudicial "master plan" runs too much risk either of injustice or of wholesale disaster. Over-all blueprints do not allow enough margin for failures and costs and discounts. "Piecemeal engineering" on an experimental and exploratory basis, to use Karl Popper's term for it, is safer because it is more flexible and pluralistic.[17]

Utopian biology, in the sense of embracing a prefabricated *system* for prefabricated human beings according to an ideal model, no matter how humane and disinterested it might be, is exactly what we ought to avoid as pretentious and fanatical. Giving it the sanction of "God's will" or "man's right" or "historical inevitability" only adds to its dangers; this is the arrogance of *hubris* that the Greeks portrayed so shrewdly in their tragic plays. J. D. Bernal, the English

Marxist, reveals it in a characteristically ideological fashion by his overstatement that natural man is now at a dead end and artificial man represents a new evolutionary stage.[18] This kind of sweeping, question-begging talk must be sedulously avoided, weeded out. We may hope that it won't prevail, because of the generally pragmatic wisdom of human beings.

Margaret Mead once recommended "Chairs of the Future" for our universities.[19] A few such chairs have actually been established, but up to this point with only uneven success. Some of them, alas, have dried up in the most woeful academic undaringness. More unfortunately we can see a tendency to cut back on the provision of training for new medical scientists. In 1973 federal support for grants was only $300 million annually—a minuscule one-half of 1 per cent of what we spend on welfare or for the armed services. The military expense is to protect us against a possible danger. Why, then, less than 1 per cent as much for the certain dangers which are sure to kill *millions* of people if we don't outwit them? The answer, of course, lies in what Francis Bacon called "purblindness"—shortsightedness. This is more the malady of politicians than of the *polis* itself.

There are many ways of looking at the options before us and many attitudes among those whose well-being is at stake. But there is no reason for despair, as experience has shown; out of the variety of our American life the most living unities are born. Said Heraclitus *circa* 500 B.C. (*Fragments* 98–99): "Opposition brings concord. Out of discord comes the fairest harmony. It is by disease that health is pleasant; by evil that good is pleasant; by hunger, satiety; by weariness, rest."

REFERENCES

(Full first names used only when needed
to avoid confusion.)

Author's Note

[1] "Where Is Biology Taking Us?" *Science*, 155 (1967), 429–33. Morison forecasts several basic changes in the family as well as in sex mores.

[2] *Chance and Necessity*. New York: Alfred A. Knopf, 1971, p. 175.

[3] Editorial, *The New Yorker*, 36 (March 5, 1960), 27.

[4] "Humanistic Biology," *American Scholar*, 34 (1965), 179.

[5] P. Medawar, *Journal of the Mt. Sinai Hospital, New York*, 36 (1969), 193.

[6] "Keeping People Alive," *Morals and Medicine*, ed. Archie Clow. New York: Oxford University Press, 1971, p. 10.

[7] S. Kleegman and S. Kaufman, *Infertility in Women*. Philadelphia: F. A. Davis Company, 1966, preface.

Some Ideas

[1] A. Toffler, *Future Shock*. New York: Random House, 1970, p. 172.

[2] *Inventing the Future*. New York: Alfred A. Knopf, 1964, p. 207.

[3] J. McHale, *The Future of the Future*. New York: George Braziller, 1969, p. 119.

[4] C. Remington, "An Experimental Study of Man's Genetic Relationship to Great Apes, by Means of Interspecific Hybridization," *Experimentation with Human Beings*, ed. J. Katz. New York: Russell Sage Foundation, 1972, pp. 461–64.

[5] *So Human an Animal*. New York: Charles Scribner's Sons, 1968, p. 106.

[6] *Hearings*, Committee on Government Operations, U. S. Senate, Joint Res. 145, Establishment of a National Com-

mission on Health, Science and Society, March 7–28, April 2, 1968, p. 40.

[7] *Genetics and the Future of Man*, ed., J. Roslansky. Amsterdam: North-Holland Publishing Company, 1966, p. 46.

[8] F. Ayd, Jr., "Fetology: Medical and Ethical Implications," *Annals of the New York Academy of Sciences*, 169 (January 21, 1970), 376–82.

[9] G. Taylor, *The Biological Time Bomb*. New York: World Publishing Company, 1968, p. 10.

[10] Editorial, *Nature*, 221 (1969), 613.

[11] *Eugenics and Science*, 35 (June 1972), 7.

[12] Quoted by C. Rivers, "Grave New World," *Saturday Review*, 55 (April 8, 1972), 23–27.

[13] *Hearings*, op. cit., p. 48.

[14] *Abortion in the United States*. New York: Paul B. Hoeber, 1958, p. 118.

[15] N. Eastman and L. Hellman, *Williams' Obstetrics*. New York: Appleton-Century-Crofts, 1961, p. 337.

[16] E. Peck, *The Baby Trap*. New York: Pinnacle Books, 1971, p. 17.

[17] "Physicians, Patients and Society: Some New Tensions in Medical Ethics," *Human Aspects of Biomedical Intervention*, ed. E. Mendelsohn, J. Swazey, and I. Taviss. Cambridge, Mass.: Harvard University Press, 1971, p. 78.

[18] "Human Evolution: Past and Future," *Genetics, Paleontology and Evolution*, ed. G. Jepson, G. Simpson, and E. Mayr. New York: Atheneum Publishers, 1963, p. 405.

[19] E. Mayr, "The Nature of the Darwinian Revolution," *Science*, 176 (June 2, 1972), 981–89.

[20] "Will Society Be Prepared?" *Science*, 157 (1967), 633.

[21] R. Dubos, "Credo of a Biologist," *Journal of Religion and Health*, 10 (1971), 313–23.

[22] G. Feinberg, *The Promethean Project*. Garden City, N.Y.: Doubleday & Company, 1969, p. 114.

[23] *The Phenomenon of Man*, intro. by J. Huxley. New York: Harper & Brothers, 1959, p. 279.

[24] *Hearings*, op. cit., p. 67.

[25] F. Burnet, "Men or Molecules: A Tilt at Molecular Biology," *Lancet*, 1 (1966), 37–39. For a full dress exposition of his views, see his *Dominant Mammal*. New York: St. Martin's Press, 1971.

[26] E. Boggs, "Choice or Chance: Some Maternal Reflections on the Prospects for New Reproductive Technologies," p. 4, a paper read at a symposium, "Choices on Our Conscience," sponsored by the Joseph P. Kennedy, Jr. Foundation, Washington, D.C., October 16, 1971.

[27] *Journal of the American Medical Association*, 220 (1972), 721.

[28] S. Hecht and M. Lappe (letter to the editor), "Moratorium on Human Zygote Implantation," *New England Journal of Medicine*, 287 (September 28, 1972), 672.

[29] Constance Holden, "World Ethics Body Proposed," *Science*, 177 (September 29, 1972), 1174.

[30] "Interests of Society?" Washington *Post*, October 21, 1967, A13.

[31] *Hearings*, op. cit., p. 59.

[32] Garden City, N.Y.: Doubleday & Company, 1966, p. 223. In this connection see E. Casteen, *The Case for Compulsory Birth Control*. Englewood Cliffs, N.J.: Prentice-Hall, 1971.

[33] D. Ingle, "Genetic Basis of Individuality and of Social Problems," *Zygon*, 6 (1971), 183.

[34] A. Shaw, "Doctor, Do We Have a Choice?" New York *Times Magazine*, January 30, 1972, 44.

[35] Th. Dobzhansky, "Man and Natural Selection," *American Scientist*, 49 (1961), 285–99.

[36] *On Law and Justice*. Cambridge, Mass.: Harvard University Press, 1945, p. 155.

[37] "Abortion and the Slippery Slope," *Dissent*, 1972, 641–43.

[38] For example, P. Ramsey, *Fabricated Man*. New Haven, Conn.: Yale University Press, 1971, *passim*.

[39] W. Gaylin, "We Have the Aweful Knowledge to Make Exact Copies of Human Beings," New York *Times Magazine*, March 5, 1972, 49.

[40] E. Kal (letter to the editor), *Journal of the American Medical Association*, 221 (September 18, 1972), 1409.

[41] *Biology and Man*. New York: Harcourt, Brace & World, 1969, p. 130.

[42] Joseph Fletcher, "American Pragmatism and the Problem of Theological Ethics," *Buffalo Studies* (State University of New York), 4 (1968), 69–85.

[43] "Better Genes for Tomorrow," *The Population Crisis and the Use of World Resources*, ed., Stuart Mudd. The Hague: W. Junk, 1964, p. 308.

Some Facts

[1] *Journal of the American Medical Association*, 220 (1972), 1356.

[2] Much help here was found in Anne McLaren, "Biological Regulation of Reproduction," *The Family and Its Future*, ed., K. Elliot. London: J. & A. Churchill, 1970, pp. 101–16 (Ciba Foundation symposium). Dr. McLaren includes adoption in her list, but it has no place there because it is not reproduction, although a genuine form of parenting. She also fails to include nuclear transplants; cloning is reproduction, although it is asexual. Another typology is set out in J. McCullough, *Genetic Engineering*, Science Research Division, Library of Congress, U. S. Government Printing Office, November 1972, pp. 14–29. The most comprehensive and scientific one, but not for popular reading, is J. Lederberg's in *Challenging Biological Problems*, ed., J. Behnke, the twenty-fifth anniversary volume of the American Institute of Biological Sciences (Oxford University Press, 1972, pp. 16–17).

[3] C. Westoff, "The Modernization of U. S. Contraceptive Practice," *Family Planning Perspectives*, 4 (July 1972), 11.

[4] Reported in *Science News*, 100 (October 30, 1971), 299.

[5] C. Carter, J. Roberts, K. Evans, "Genetic Clinic: A Follow-Up," *Lancet*, 1 (1971), 281–85.

[6] C. Leonard, G. Chase, B. Childs, "Genetic Counseling:

A Consumer's View," *New England Journal of Medicine*, 287 (1972), 433–39.

[7] M. Kaback and J. O'Brien, "Tay-Sachs: Prototype for Prevention of Genetic Disease," *Hospital Practice*, March 1973, 115–16.

[8] "The Family Secret" (a special report), *Ladies' Home Journal*, 89 (September 1972), 86–92, 208.

[9] T. Friedman and R. Roblin, "Gene Therapy for Human Genetic Disease?" *Science*, 175 (March 3, 1972), 949–54.

[10] D. Wooldridge, *Mechanical Man: The Physical Basis of Intelligent Life*. New York: McGraw-Hill Book Co., 1968, p. 81.

[11] A. Motulsky, G. Fraser, J. Felsenstein, "Public Health and Long-Term Genetic Implications of Intrauterine Diagnosis and Selective Abortion," *Birth Defects: Original Articles Series*, Medical College of Virginia, 7 (April 1971), 23.

[12] Op. cit., p. 169.

[13] See the thesis of A. Jansen, "How Much Can We Boost I.Q. and Intellectual Achievement?" *Harvard Education Review*, 39 (1969), 533–43.

[14] New York *Times*, August 8, 1972, 1 and 67.

Some Doubts

[1] M. Graubard, "The Frankenstein Syndrome: Man's Ambivalent Attitude to Knowledge and Power," *Perspectives in Biology and Medicine*, 10 (1967), 419–33.

[2] For example, see *Values and the Future*, K. Baier and N. Rescher, eds. New York: The Macmillan Co., 1969, pp. 133–47.

[3] *The Human Agenda*. New York: Simon & Schuster, 1972, pp. 197–231.

[4] L. Kass, "New Beginnings in Life," *The New Genetics and the Future of Man*, ed., Michael Hamilton. Grand Rapids, Mich.: Wm. B. Eerdmans Publishing Company, 1972, pp. 53–63.

[5] G. Wolstenholme, *Man and His Future*. Boston: Little,

Brown and Company, 1963, pp. 284–97 (Ciba Foundation symposium).

[6] "A Psychological View of Religion in the 1970s," *Bulletin of the Menninger Clinic*, 35 (1971), 77–97.

[7] J. Littlefield, quoted by B. Kramer, *The Wall Street Journal*, 168 (October 14, 1966), 1 and 13.

[8] L. Kass, op. cit., p. 55.

[9] K. Ludmerer, *Genetics and American Society*. Baltimore: The Johns Hopkins University Press, 1972, pp. 116–17.

[10] L. Kass, op. cit., p. 39.

[11] "Portents for a Genetic Engineering," *Journal of Heredity*, 56 (1965), 197–202.

[12] Quoted in A. Rosenfeld, *The Second Genesis*. Englewood Cliffs, N.J.: Prentice-Hall, 1969, p. 158.

[13] *Physical Control of the Mind*. New York: Harper & Row, 1969, p. 38.

[14] *Abortion: The Personal Dilemma*. London: The Paternoster Press, 1972, p. 124.

[15] P. Ramsey, "Shall We 'Reproduce'?" *Journal of the American Medical Association*, 220 (1972), 1347.

[16] Ibid., p. 1348.

[17] See the objections listed and discussed in Joseph Fletcher, *Morals and Medicine*. Boston: Beacon Press, 1960 (Princeton University Press, 1954), esp. pp. 106–40.

[18] See his *Adam's New Rib*. New York: Harcourt Brace Jovanovich, 1972, p. 90. Also his *Utopian Motherhood*. Garden City, N.Y.: Doubleday & Company, 1970.

[19] P. Ramsey, *Fabricated Man*. New Haven, Conn.: Yale University Press, 1970, p. 40.

[20] P. Ramsey, *The Patient as Person*. New Haven, Conn.: Yale University Press, 1970, p. 2.

[21] R. G. Gorney, *The Human Agenda*, op. cit., p. 201.

[22] L. Kass, "Freedom, Coercion and Asexual Reproduction," *Experimentation with Human Beings*, op. cit., p. 979.

[23] E. Messenger, *Evolution and Theology*. London: Burns, Oates & Washbourne, 1931.

[24] P. Ramsey, "The Ethics of a Cottage Industry in an Age of Community and Research Medicine," *New Eng-*

land Journal of Medicine, 284 (April 1, 1971), 703; and editorial, 727.

25 Quoted in G. Taylor, op. cit., p. 225.

26 V. Zorba in *The Guardian Weekly*, December 13, 1969, 6.

27 *Britannica Book of the Year 1964.* Chicago: Encyclopedia Britannica, Inc., pp. 499–500.

28 Quoted in A. Rosenfeld, op. cit., p. 145.

29 L. Kass, "New Beginnings in Life," op. cit., p. 60.

30 Quoted in E. Torrey, "Ethical Issues in Future Medicine," *Toward Century 21*, ed. C. Wallia. New York: Basic Books, 1970, p. 34.

31 B. Webb, O.S.B., *Catholic Medical Quarterly*, 24 (October 1972), 69–75.

32 "Prospect for Genetic Intervention in Man," reprinted from *Science* in *Genetic Engineering*, op. cit., pp. 78–85.

Some Issues

1 *Science*, 162 (1968), 1243–48; elaborated in Hardin's *Exploring New Ethics for Survival: The Voyage of the Spaceship Beagle.* New York: The Viking Press, 1972, pp. 250–68.

2 John Fletcher, "The Brink: The Parent-Child Bond in the Genetic Revolution," *Theological Studies* 33 (September 1972), 476–78.

3 Joseph Fletcher, "Virtue as a Predicate," *The Monist*, 54 (1970), 66–85, and his *Moral Responsibility*. Philadelphia: Westminster Press, 1967, pp. 29–41.

4 P. Ramsey, *Fabricated Man*, op. cit., p. 30.

5 R. Gardner, *Abortion: A Personal Dilemma*, op. cit., p. 106.

6 "Some Thoughts on the Ethics of Reproductive Technology," *Choices on Our Conscience*, Kennedy Foundation, op. cit.

7 W. Henley, *New Zealand Medical Journal*, 68 (1966), 144.

8 I. Brant, *The Bill of Rights*. New York: The New American Library, 1965.

[9] "Eugenics and Religion," *Eugenics Review*, 60 (1968), 92–98.

[10] "Humanizing the Earth," *Science*, 179 (1973), 769–72.

[11] J. Mayr, "Decision Making in the Biological Field," *Perspectives in Biology and Medicine*, 16 (1972), 36–50.

[12] *The Future of Man*, op. cit., p. 100.

[13] *Speculation: Essays in Humanism and the Philosophy of Art*. New York: Harcourt, Brace & Company, 1946, p. 11.

[14] *Sex, Man and Society*. New York: G. P. Putnam's Sons, 1969.

[15] *Man and People*. New York: W. W. Norton & Company, 1957.

[16] "Life and the Right to Life," *Ethical Issues in Human Genetics*, eds., B. Hilton, D. Callahan, M. Harris, P. Condliffe, B. Berkley. New York: Plenum Press, 1973, p. 182.

[17] J. Noonan, ed. *The Morality of Abortion*. Cambridge, Mass.: Harvard University Press, 1970, p. xvii.

[18] See Joseph Fletcher, *Situation Ethics*. Philadelphia: Westminster Press, 1966, p. 38.

[19] *Humanly Possible*. New York: Saturday Review Press, 1973, p. 88.

[20] *Abortion in a Changing World*, ed., R. Hall. New York: Columbia University Press, 1970, Vol. 2.

[21] *Humanly Possible*, op. cit., pp. 46 and 66.

[22] Ibid., p. 56.

[23] See Joseph Fletcher, *Morals and Medicine*, op. cit., pp. 116–22.

Some Answers

[1] G. Dunstan, *Morals and Medicine*, ed., Archie Clow, op. cit., p. 67.

[2] "Genetic Engineering," *Engineering and Science*, 35 (June 1972), 7.

[3] "A New Ethic for Medicine and Society," *California Medicine*, 113 (September 1970), 67–68.

[4] See H. Muller, "Human Evolution by Voluntary Choice of Germ Plasm," *Science*, 134 (September 8, 1961), 643–49 for a suggestive exposition.

[5] In a play by J. Costigan, *Baby Want a Kiss?*

[6] *Hospital Tribune*, 7:14 (April 9, 1973), 1, 24.

[7] Quoted by E. Grossman, "The Obsolescent Mother," *Atlantic Monthly*, 227 (May 1971), 39–50.

[8] Joseph Fletcher, in *Marriage: For and Against*, intro. by H. Hart. New York: Hart Publishing Co., 1972, p. 205.

[9] *Future Shock*, op. cit., 208.

[10] S. Behrman, in Behrman and Kistner, *Progress in Infertility*. Boston: Little, Brown and Company, 1967.

[11] *The Promethean Project*. Garden City, N.Y.: Doubleday & Company, 1969, pp. 203–5.

[12] *The Foreseeable Future*. New York: The Viking Press, 1960, p. 98.

[13] *The Biocrats*. New York: McGraw-Hill Book Co., 1970, p. 98.

[14] R. Francoeur, *Adam's New Rib*, op. cit., pp. 221–24.

[15] In *The Place of Value in a World of Facts*, ed., A. Tiselius and S. Nilsson. New York and London: John Wiley & Sons, 1971.

[16] *Bioethics: Bridge to the Future*. Englewood Cliffs, N.J.: Prentice-Hall, 1971, p. 70.

[17] *The Use of Fetuses and Fetal Material for Research*. London: Her Majesty's Stationery Office, 1972.

[18] *Exploring New Ethics for Survival*. New York: The Viking Press, 1972, pp. 260–62.

[19] F. Grad, "Legislative Responses to the New Biology: Limits and Possibilities," *U.C.L.A. Law Review*, 15 (February 1968), 486.

[20] Quoted by A. Rosenfeld, op. cit., p. 161.

[21] "Birth Defects," *Humanistic Perspectives in Medical Ethics*, ed., M. Visscher. London: Pemberton Publishing Co., 1972, p. 207.

Some Hopes

[1] *On Aggression*. New York: Bantam Books, 1967, p. 221.

[2] *The Genetic Code*. New York: Orion Press, 1962, p. 175.

[3] *Inventing the Future*, op. cit., p. 104.

[4] Joseph Fletcher, "Medicine's Scientific Developments and Resulting Ethical Problems," *Dialogue in Medicine and Theology*, ed., D. White. New York: Abingdon Press, 1967, p. 150.

[5] *The Scientific Outlook*. New York: W. W. Norton & Co., 1972, p. 254. This is a lecture given at Columbia University in 1929.

[6] New York: George Braziller, 1967.

[7] In *The Control of Human Heredity and Evolution*, ed. T. Sonneborn. New York: The Macmillan Co., 1965, p. 81.

[8] "Reflections on Law and Experimental Medicine," *U.C.L.A. Law Review*, 15 (1968), 440.

[9] Op. cit., pp. 580–89.

[10] *The Family and the Future*, op. cit., p. 112.

[11] R. Francoeur, *Utopian Motherhood*, op. cit., p. 8.

[12] *Population and the American Future*, op. cit., pp. 263–66.

[13] Op. cit., p. vii.

[14] "Directed Genetic Change: Perspectives for Molecular Genetics," *The Control of Human Heredity and Evolution*, op. cit., p. 3.

[15] *Humanly Possible*, op. cit., p. 153.

[16] Editorial, *Science*, 172 (April 9, 1971), 11.

[17] *The Open Society and Its Enemies*. Princeton, N.J.: Princeton University Press, 1950, p. 158.

[18] *The World, the Flesh and the Devil*. London: Jonathan Cape, Ltd., 1970.

[19] *Science*, 126 (1957), 960.